Crushing the Peanut

Food Allergy Life before and after Oral Immunotherapy

by Katy Patrick

Cover design by Archangel Ink, LLC www.archangelink.com
Editing by Katie Chambers www.tutorwithkatie.org
Author photograph by Ian McCalister www.ianmccalister.com
Formatting by Nerdy Wordsmith Ink www.nerdywordsmith.com

Nothing in this book is intended as a substitute for the medical advice of physicians. The reader should regularly consult a physician in matters relating to his/her health and particularly with respect to any symptoms that may require diagnosis or medical attention. In regards to all food allergy, oral immunotherapy and other health dialogue in this story, the author's words and experiences are not intended to be a "how-to" but rather an accounting of "how-it-felt-to" from the author's perspective.

ISBN: 1543214789
ISBN-13: 978-1543214789

TABLE OF CONTENTS

Foreword 1

Introduction 6

Chapter 1 - First Touch 12

Chapter 2 - First Test 19

Chapter 3 - First Bite 27

Chapter 4 - Twice Bitten 38

Chapter 5 - First and Last School 48

Chapter 6 - Third Bite 62

Chapter 7 - Last Chance to Outgrow 74

Chapter 8 - Fourth and Fifth Bites 84

Chapter 9 - Searching and Researching 96

Chapter 10 - Consultations 109

Chapter 11 - A Food Challenge 119

Chapter 12 - Starting Peanut OIT 131

Chapter 13 - Updosing Appointments 141

Chapter 14 - Traveling 152

Chapter 15 - OIT with a Teen 162

Chapter 16 - Graduating to Maintenance 171

Chapter 17 - Life After OIT 182

Acknowledgments 188

References 191

FOREWORD

This is a glimpse into a food allergy mom's heart and soul. If you are a parent, a loved one, or a friend of someone with a life-threatening food allergy, I invite you to sit a spell with me. I am not alone in having a food allergy story to tell, but this is the drama that played out inside my heart and head over the past 17 years, which I have spilled onto these pages.

My name is Katy and I live, love, and parent with an amazing dad who is also my best friend and partner, Kurt. We are mom and dad to one of the estimated 15 million Americans who have food allergies. There are eight foods that cause most allergic reactions: peanuts, tree nuts, eggs, milk, soy, fish, shellfish and wheat. Approximately three million of those allergic in the United States are allergic to peanuts. A Food Allergy Research & Education (FARE) funded study indicated that between 1997 and 2008, peanut allergy among children more than tripled.

My son, Alex, is a part of that unexplained, scary statistic of tripled peanut allergies, but he doesn't just have any peanut allergy, he has peanut anaphylaxis, which means his allergy is life-threatening. If he ingests peanuts and doesn't get treatment quickly, Alex's body can shut down, and he can die.

Alex got in early on the food allergy population surge as he first reacted to peanuts visibly in 2000, via contact with a toy as an infant at five months old. It became apparent later that Alex had exhibited allergic symptoms in the months before he ever touched that peanut butter smeared toy.

For sixteen years, we lived in fear for the future, a fear that accompanies any life-threatening food allergy diagnosis. Then in 2014, I found what sounded like a miracle, OIT. OIT is the acronym for Oral Immunotherapy. If you got this book, you might know what OIT entails. If not, the OIT101[1] website has a wealth of research, data, and support for those interested in OIT.

The OIT101 website explains, "OIT is a 'social and emotional cure' as a food allergy treatment. Oral Immunotherapy desensitizes children & adults to their food allergens. By consuming the allergen regularly, in increasing amounts under the care of a board-certified allergist, patients' immune systems adapt to the allergen that formerly would have caused a life-threatening anaphylactic reaction. Desensitized patients are still allergic. They consume their allergen regularly to maintain desensitization. We say it's a 'social cure' because it eliminates social exclusion due to food allergies and the many social confrontations that come from questioning every bite of food. We say it's an 'emotional cure' because it eliminates fear of food, and of feeling different or left out from peers" (OIT101, 2016a).

This story on my son's peanut allergy and OIT journey is not a how to guide, nor is it a debate or a propaganda piece to convince anyone on what they should or shouldn't do about a food allergy. OIT is not for everyone; while it has success rates of over 85%, it's a hard thing to consider doing, and it is not available everywhere. It's a big step to wrap your head and mind around introducing, even in minute amounts, the allergen you've been avoiding for yourself or your child for years. Not everyone can travel to get this treatment. Unfortunately, there are still allergists who do not refer patients to OIT even though it is researched and performed by their own board-certified peers. OIT should only be done under the consultation and care of a board certified OIT trained allergist familiar with the protocols deemed safe and effective in trials and practice for over a decade.

Here, I juxtapose our 16 years of surviving a peanut allergy with the contrast of living after my son's Oral Immunotherapy for peanut allergy. If you have OIT specific questions, if you want to see peer reviewed medical research, if you are looking for a listing of private practice OIT allergists, or you want to give OIT a look if you've never heard of it, then I encourage you to head to OIT101.

The OIT101 website was built and is maintained by a dedicated group of food allergy parents who were instrumental in bringing awareness to parents of food allergic kids that OIT was available by private practice allergists. This group shared via Facebook in the years prior to their website forming in 2016. The history of OIT is detailed on their webpage and is a long and fascinating read.

I do not personally know any of the food allergy parents that formed these groups, but I am forever grateful to have stumbled across their OIT101 Facebook page[2] in 2015 and their Private Practice OIT page[3] in 2016. They also maintain Facebook pages for OIT in Canada[4], in the United Kingdom[5] and Australia[6] at this time. I was never able to fully turn away from the idea of OIT once I read about and researched the protocol. In Oral Immunotherapy, I saw a steady flicker of light at the end of a suffocating tunnel of food avoidance.

My goal is to be transparent and share what parenting a child with a life-threatening food allergy from childhood into teen years was like. And, then to share what life was like after undergoing and graduating from Oral Immunotherapy. My goal in sharing is both personal and altruistic. Personally, I need to get this story that roams around the halls of my head into a concise narrative. I throw tidbits out at different interested people one bit at a time, but my experience needs a resting place. I need to corral all the allergy years and give them a home and some closure.

Altruistically, my goal is twofold. First, I hope others will understand and appreciate the hardships of raising a child while avoiding a food allergen. Second, I hope that at least one person who reads this story decides to give OIT a look sooner rather than later. Or maybe he or she will share OIT with one food allergic person that he or she knows. If that happens, then being vulnerable on these pages will all have been worth it. It was a group of strangers that gave the gift of OIT to me, so I hope to give the same gift to another stranger affected by food allergy.

Additionally, I also want to physically give OIT access to others. Right now, OIT is not available everywhere. As of this writing, there are over 70 vetted board certified private practice OIT allergists in the United States. That is not a lot compared to the many food allergy sufferers looking for hope. Many families travel great distances, even from overseas, to visit a private practice OIT doctor. I want to help make the limited access less of a burden for others.

I pledge to donate half of the proceeds from this book to help others access OIT, in whatever form that takes. My donation may help other allergists receive the training and education needed to practice OIT, or my donation may go to help patients pay for the cost of traveling to an OIT doctor, or my donation may help OIT101 carry out their mission of spreading awareness and transforming lives. There is a non-profit formed to fund the mission of the OIT101 website, OIT Works, Inc. That is the legal entity that proceeds will fund. I am committed to helping others access OIT.

I don't want to profit from our food allergy story. Instead, I want our story to be a part of changing food allergy lives. The other half of the proceeds of this book will go to my son, Alex, for him to put toward the change he wants to see in the world. This is his story through my eyes. By reading, you are helping me pay forward the gift that OIT has been in my son's life. Thank you.

INTRODUCTION

I am a bit of a nutcase, both literally and figuratively. A nut, the peanut, drove me crazy and down into some deep mental caverns over the years. While I am recovering from the insanity, fear, and anxiety of having a child with a life-threatening food allergy, I now celebrate a free-from-fear, thriving 17-year-old son who used to be deathly allergic to peanuts and is now miraculously "bite-safe" to those same nuts.

Until this past year, I was merely surviving, living in fear with the reality of my son's allergy. I was that stereotypical nutty (pun intended), obsessive compulsive, anxiety riddled mom of a peanut allergic child. You might have embraced in sympathy someone like me in your community, or you might have run away confused not understanding what fueled that crazy allergy parent, or you might see yourself in me. For over a decade and a half, fear was my ally and my taskmaster. It kept Alex safe and alive and me at the top of my protector game.

During Alex's 16th year, I broke out of that impossible role, and instead, I experienced a year of hope and a future life of freedom that still feels surreal today. I hope something I share inspires you to realize there is hope for the person whom you care about with a life-threatening food allergy. I hope you also see on these pages that childhood with a food allergy can be a beautiful thing despite the limitations and the fear. I will share things that we wouldn't have in our lives, choices we would not have made, if not for Alex having a peanut allergy. For those choices, I am forever grateful that he was born allergic.

Our lives have come full circle with the peanut. Alex was born in 1999 in Georgia, one of several states with a city claiming to be the peanut capital of the world. The allergy community over the past 17 years has gone from one recommendation concerning infants and pregnant mothers to another. At times, they recommended pregnant mothers and babies should be exposed to peanuts. At other times, the recommendation has swung to the other side of the spectrum: pregnant mothers and babies should practice strict avoidance if there is a risk of allergy.

Recently, several groups including the American Academy of Pediatrics (AAP) and the National Institute of Allergy and Infectious Diseases (NIAID) announced that guidelines now recommend infants at high risk of peanut allergy be introduced to peanuts at 4 to 6 months of age due to the promising results from the Learning Early About Peanut allergy (LEAP) trial over the past five years. Additionally, the NIAID produced a brochure that gives clarity to these new peanut introduction guidelines. The publication details how to tell which infants are at risk and who might need testing before introducing peanut foods into their diet (2017).

My head has spun over the years at the back and forth of what is the 'right' thing to do to prevent your kid from having a peanut allergy. I don't know that I will ever know why Alex was allergic to peanuts or if I could have prevented it by doing anything differently. I do know that our three children born after Alex are not allergic to peanuts or any other foods. I know what I did differently with them, but what I did differently doesn't always mesh with the researched recommendations. In the end, it is just my little four subject sample study, fallible and statistically unsound. It would be egregious for me to claim I know why my other kids aren't allergic and Alex is, but I do speculate.

My speculations include genetics, my eating habits, his environment, my gluten intolerance, and exposure to vaccinations and antibiotics. While I will never know, I speculate over the many factors that could have contributed to this.

The twists of fate that marked Alex's immune system and triggered it to attack peanuts are unknown. We learned after Alex was diagnosed that Alex's dad, Kurt, used to get diaper rashes as a toddler after eating peanut butter. Perhaps Alex inherited a genetic predisposition to peanut allergy from his dad? Kurt and I have a line of grandmothers and relatives that were allergic to everything from cats, hazelnuts, pecans, and brazil nuts to environmental allergens. Perhaps that genetic history played a role?

I was a healthy eater during pregnancy, but I could also make questionable eating choices. Continuing an odd tradition I learned as a teenager, I would often down a glass bottle of coke filled with a snack size bag of peanuts on road trips to my parent's house. During my whole pregnancy with Alex and while breastfeeding him, both the peanut and its butter were a staple in my diet. Perhaps, my constant peanut consumption gave Alex an overdose of the nut and sensitized him in utero. There are new guidelines, which I mentioned, for introducing peanut to infants at risk, but there are not published recommended guidelines yet for pregnant mothers to either ingest or avoid peanut products during their pregnancy. Hopefully, in the future, guidelines for pregnant mothers will give more clarity to this piece of the puzzle.

Alex didn't live in a sterile environment, so it might seem unlikely for the "hygiene hypothesis" of allergy and autoimmune disorders to affect him. But Alex was born in the United States, a highly developed country where this hypothesis could play a role in allergy. The hygiene hypotheses states that lack of early childhood exposure to different infectious agents, microorganisms, and parasites increases chances of allergy because the immune system doesn't develop naturally. Maybe Alex's immune system didn't develop properly due to his environment. The kink in this theory is that he was born allergic to peanuts before the hygiene hypothesis or environment could affect his immune system.

I learned in 2005 that I was gluten intolerant. Maybe this condition damaged my intestinal tract and affected absorption of peanut proteins into my bloodstream. Did this affect how I passed them on to my child while I was pregnant or when he was still breastfeeding?

Alex had all his vaccinations on schedule. He was exposed to vaccines at birth and in the first months of his life. Heather Fraser (2015), in her book, *The Peanut Allergy Epidemic (2nd Edition)*, raises concerns about vaccine mechanisms causing cross reactivity to peanuts. She details studies and suggests findings that point to vaccines contributing to the rise in peanut allergy. It's a compelling book. So, perhaps these handful of vaccines affected Alex?

Alex had a few rounds of antibiotics as a young infant for ear infections and a bacterial infection. Perhaps that messed with his gut microbiome which in turn affected his immune systems development or sensitization to peanuts?

I could go on for pages on the what ifs. Was it environmental factors or genetics? I don't hold my breath that I'll ever know. For whatever reasons, Alex was anaphylactic to peanuts.

Regardless, we learned to survive living with a peanut allergy. Our lives handling this peanut allergy started in Georgia, and even though we now live in a different state, we ironically found his food allergy salvation back in Georgia at Freedom Allergy private practice OIT. For OIT, we put Alex in the hands and care of a man that is a superhero disguised as an allergist in a shirt and tie. He is a board certified private practice OIT allergist who, like a small group of other pioneering allergists around the United States, is banishing fear and anxiety and giving those who are allergic back their lives. I send love, a hug, and my unending gratitude to Dr. Agrawal, Danielle, and his staff who make dreams come true. Here's the peanut allergy story in our family; how we went from surviving to thriving and crushed the peanut's effect on our lives.

CHAPTER 1 - FIRST TOUCH

I never got to experience the joy of parenting without extreme anxiety. With fear constantly lurking, its heavy cloak on my shoulders, its jade colored glasses skewing my view, my parenting journey was devoid of the normal letting go that happens as your child ages, has milestones, and ventures out into the world.

Alex made Kurt and me parents in the fall of 1999. He was a full term, healthy seven pound baby with a sunny disposition except for bouts of colic and constant eczema that made him uncomfortable. I breastfed him exclusively until he could sit up and displayed signs he was ready for solid foods. In the first few months of his life, I had normal anxiety: figuring out how to feed and calm him and navigating sleep and life with a baby needing me twenty-four hours. But I didn't really fear for his life. I was awash in the blissful hormone of oxytocin, and life as a new mother was calm.

Sure, I experienced normal anxiety at first, but the deathly fear took hold within a few months. Alex first exhibited a reaction to peanuts at about five months. Before he had tried solids, before he could sit up, before he could crawl, before I ever worried about what he could stumble and cut his head upon, before I lunged to stop him from putting a marble in his mouth, I had a bigger beast to contend with: worrying what could touch Alex that had peanuts in it.

The fear all started on what should have been a fun journey with our neighbors. Since this was the year 2000, connecting with other parents still took a lot of physical face time. The online spaces for meeting, socializing, and discussing we have today did not exist. Thus, I had to get out of my pajamas and overcome more hurdles than just having an internet connection in order to find another parent to connect with as a friend. Whom I bonded with and reached out to depended a lot on physical location. Living in a sprawling Atlanta suburb with an infant that hated riding in the car, I was a pretty static dot on the map.

I met Pam two doors down. She had two toddler boys and worked as a baby nurse in a local hospital Labor and Delivery unit. She gave me confidence in dealing with belly buttons and diapers and a myriad of other unknown baby questions. With her next door, I didn't feel as alone in my long winter days with my baby. I envisioned Alex as a toddler and a child playing with these slightly older boys, roaming, exploring, and forming childhood bonds. Pam and I bonded over mundane moments: matching Halloween costumes, breastfeeding, kids sipping blue kool-aid, swims in her in-law's pool, more afternoons of cartoons than I'd watched since I was a kid, all peppered with kid interrupted conversations.

When Alex was 5 months old in the spring of 2000, we went to a small-town stock car race with Pam's family. Their hobby of racing cars had turned into a family business, and they invited us to see them race a car in a show south of Atlanta. Stock car racing was completely foreign to me, but I was a stay-at-home mom looking for connections, and the closest human to me in those early months was my neighbor.

So, we packed up the car and headed out for the drive south to watch our neighbors race with Alex sleeping as we went. It was stereotypical of what you might think of a stock car race: Loud. Dusty. Testosterone filled. The fuel in the air sent a stinging tang to my nostrils. It was a do-it-yourself car lover's paradise. Marveling at this hobby and passion that had become bigger than folk's weekend projects and garages, I glanced around at the place filled with cars and the crews that went with them.

I carried Alex around all day in a baby carrier on my chest or a sling on my shoulder. I stopped periodically to nurse him in the quiet of the racing trailer, or our car, or in a folding chair set up near the group. Since it wasn't an environment conducive to allowing a baby to play or sleep on the ground, I tired of holding him as the day went on. That afternoon, to stretch my tired arms and back, I set him down on a blanket on the floor of the racing trailer with Pam's toddlers nearby and handed him a toy from the kid debris on the floor. I remember he had on a white footed onesie of some sort, covered in a baby bear pattern with long sleeves. I imagine I'd covered every inch of his skin in clothing to keep him warm and from getting dirty at the racetrack.

The toy I handed him was a silver rattle; I chose it thinking that he could mouth on the cool metal and soothe his swollen gums. Alex couldn't sit up yet, and he wanted to be moving and busy all the time. I could sense frustration in his tiny body to move and communicate. Into his chubby baby hands the rattle went. The next thing I knew, his mouth and hands were red, he had welts forming around his mouth and on the backs of his hands. The welts were scattered going up his cheek and onto his forehead.

I panicked and called for Pam, my friend and nurse. In concern she asked, "What did he have, where had he been, what happened?" We searched for some insect or spider at first and saw nothing. "He was just playing here on the blanket with this rattle," I remember exclaiming.

We both looked at the rattle in my hand, and I think she made the connection before me. "Oh,'" she said, "I think Austin had this in his hand, and he's been eating a peanut butter and jelly sandwich and probably smeared peanut butter on the rattle. Lots of kids are allergic to peanuts these days, maybe Alex is allergic to peanuts and reacting to touching it on the rattle?" I whisked Alex's onesie off and panicked at the sight of the welts, which I later learned were hives, all over his torso and back. He was indeed reacting to touching and possibly mouthing the rattle that had peanut butter residue on it.

Pam got baby wipes to wipe his hands and body down, and I remember promptly nursing him while she did this. I was hoping that the magic of breastmilk could rinse away this horror. Pam was the prepared type and had a children's liquid antihistamine with her. We gave that to Alex as well. I was expecting a sudden swollen face with eyes closed shut and trouble breathing, like you see exaggerated in the movies, but that didn't happen. The hives got to a point and didn't spread much more and his breathing never changed audibly. I know Pam checked his pulse and went to see if the medics that were in the race area were prepared to help someone with a reaction. I know I abdicated decision making and looked to others for what to do and how to handle this. I remember asking where the nearest hospital was and wondering with Kurt if we should head that way.

It was terrifying sitting there nursing Alex and waiting for the hives to subside. But since I was taking my cues from Pam, I didn't feel in charge. I was not owning any responsibility for the outcome or action that needed to be taken. Kurt wasn't either. We were not prepared in any way, knowledge or otherwise, to conquer an allergic reaction. There was so much I didn't yet know or understand about anaphylactic food allergies. In this first contact reaction, I didn't feel as in charge or as concerned as I should have been. My fear was confined to the present tense dread of that moment at the race with Alex covered in welts.

Fear visited me that day but didn't become a part of my everyday horizon until about one year later when I realized the full extent of

Alex's allergy and what life would become. At the racetrack, that first taste of fear was compartmentalized into an isolated incident. I was a deer in the headlights that had dodged being struck by a car. Certainly, I was stunned with this peanut incident, but after it wore off, the pounding of my heart subsided. Alex was in the clear, and we had made it to the other side of the road.

I was either in denial or unaware of the steps I needed to take after seeing those hives on Alex's body. I didn't realize that this wasn't a fluke occurrence. As stupid as that might sound, I just didn't know I had to do anything other than ensure Alex avoided peanuts in case it happened again. Like the deer that experiences dodging a car for the first time and becomes wary of headlights, I proceeded as a parent dodging peanuts. I became aware of peanuts and didn't give Alex any peanut foods as he became a food gobbling one year old. I kept a concerned eye out because I didn't want to experience that fear again, but I didn't have full knowledge of what I was looking out for. I didn't realize that true avoidance for a true allergy was a different sort of position.

On top of that, our pediatrician had not advised me to see an allergist, even knowing about the hives incident from the rattle and knowing that Alex had eczema. The doctor was not concerned so I was not concerned either. My intuition should have known to seek further medical advice. I was inexperienced and young, and it didn't occur to me to listen to my concerns and get a second opinion.

This denial was a two-step dance I did with food allergy for about a year. For some reason, I didn't take it a step further and take him to an allergist to get educated and informed on how to deal with food allergy properly. However, I did at least conduct some research online to try and figure out how he could be contact allergic when he had never even eaten any food. There was some information pointing towards children being sensitized in utero. I felt guilty for all the JIF peanut butter that had gotten me through the hunger of my pregnancy with Alex. I vowed to never eat peanuts while pregnant again. To me, it was that simple: avoid peanuts. Testing and *EpiPens* and allergists were off my radar. Although I was gifted a warning sign in that rattle incident, the warning sign just wasn't loud enough; like the silver rattle, it was merely a tiny tinkling noise.

CHAPTER 2 - FIRST TEST

Fast forward to Alex at 17 months old (almost a year later). I was newly pregnant with my second child, and I, along with my mom and another good friend, headed that summer to Chicago for a conference. We had three adults and two toddlers on the trip. Based on my reading on exposure to allergens in utero, I was eating a completely peanut free diet and not eating many other nuts either. I was taking precautions, but without medical advice, I was winging it.

The conference in Chicago was a family friendly conference and the hotel and rooms were filled with babies, kids, and families. To avoid peanuts, Alex ate only his snacks and our food and no nuts. On day two of the conference, in a line for the bathrooms, another woman offered Alex a cookie. In the sheltered life created in the rural suburb we lived in, it wasn't often that my toddler was offered food by a stranger. He was only 17 months, and didn't go to daycare or anything similar. I was pretty much at his side always. I thought the cookies she had looked like peanut butter cookies. They had the signature crisscross fork pattern on the top. I thanked her for offering, but declined sharing, "I think he's allergic to peanuts, so we had better not have one."

Another woman in the bathroom line overheard this exchange and approached me. She was the first food allergy advocate I had ever spoken to. She said she didn't mean to intrude, but did I just say my son *might* be or *was* allergic to peanuts? I explained the rattle incident when he was an infant and our avoidance since he started eating food and saw her eyebrows rise and heard her tone change. She told her child's story of anaphylaxis, and explained to me how important it was to know the severity of the allergy and to have an *EpiPen* on hand if the allergy was life-threatening. She urged me to waste no time in seeing a pediatric allergist to get my son tested for peanut allergy. She warned, "He won't be little forever, and you can't always be watching. One day he will put something in his mouth." She made me promise to see an allergist and carry an *EpiPen* if testing proved he needed it. I felt thankful she had crossed our path. I realized I might have put Alex in danger by not being a better allergy advocate and researcher and taking him to an allergist sooner.

As soon as we got home, I broke out our list of insurance providers and found a pediatric allergist. Before the summer was over, we were in the allergist's office for a consultation. She took a detailed history of Alex's birth, skin conditions, illnesses, any history of asthma (he had none), what reactions he had had, creams and medicines he was on, etc. Then she gave her recommendation. A full panel of skin tests.

Lying down on the examination table side by side with my shirtless little boy, I held him while he got pricks for allergens all over his back. There were so many. We waited the time frame to see what reactions materialized. Results came back positive for peanuts, grasses, and dust mites.

They gave us an *EpiPen* prescription, clear directions on administering it, along with the firm and final diagnosis that Alex was severely allergic to peanuts. While we didn't have the blood lab results yet, the doctor assumed based on Alex's history and the skin test that the results would show he was anaphylactic. She advised us to proceed as if he were anaphylactic, and she would let us know if the labs showed otherwise. She recommended steps to lower Alex's exposure to dust mites and grasses and how to educate ourselves on all the likely food contamination dangers of peanuts. In addition, I learned that Alex's eczema was likely tied to his allergy. He might have been getting minute amounts of peanut exposure in my breastmilk when he was still nursing and minute amounts in cross contaminated foods that he had been eating. To further educate us, we were shown a video about food allergies and anaphylaxis as well as a video on how to administer an *EpiPen*.

The allergist did us a big favor in accurate and thorough education at that first visit even though it felt over the top at the time. The allergy videos and *EpiPen* training seemed designed more to scare us than to educate us. However, in that office was the first time I sat and thought and realized that Alex could die from his allergy. That was numbing to contemplate and sent me into a full body visceral alert state. The doctor and nurse seemed so certain that Alex would have a reaction, and we would need to use his *EpiPen*. I was skeptical. I had not yet been humbled by experiencing a full ingestion and full anaphylactic reaction. I'd seen him have hives from the rattle and seen that they went away that day at the racetrack.

The allergist advised us not to be afraid or hesitate when Alex had a reaction and needed the *EpiPen*. She said it likely would happen, that it was a when and not an if. But now, I was going to be even better at avoiding peanut products, so I wondered how Alex could possibly accidentally ingest. Peanut was just one allergen, and so many kids had several allergens, surely it wouldn't be that hard to avoid just this one. I had kept him safe thus far, and he was a grabbing toddler. Would it not just get easier to avoid as he got older? I thought food avoidance was more invincible and controllable than it is. I didn't realize how much food is in everything we do and how that would play out as Alex got older.

She continued with her clear instructions: when it happened, we couldn't hesitate, we needed to act. She assured us that the epinephrine injector was safe, that it couldn't hurt him. If we knew he had started having a reaction after eating something, and we knew the signs, then the *EpiPen* was his lifeline. We would have what we needed to stop the reaction and proceed to the emergency room. I am grateful she had us leave her office with confidence before I held that auto injector in my hand for the first time. It would have been hard to jab the device into my son's tiny thigh had

I not been coached about its safety and urgency while calmly sitting in an office instead of in the middle of an allergic reaction.

That day I got the message loud and clear that life from here on out would be different. Having an allergist's diagnosis and detailed prognosis on allergen avoidance rather than just my deductions from the rattle incident was a different world. This August day, I switched into survival mode. While I had chosen to always protect him and stay close to him, I no longer felt like this was just a parenting choice, but rather a life-threatening necessity. However, I had been protecting him secretly, privately, almost shamefully and not very well. Perhaps, I just didn't want Alex to be different and diagnosed as severely allergic; thus, I immaturely parented him that year in denial. This could have put Alex's life in danger.

I thought we had been lucky beyond measure that Alex had not experienced a life-threatening reaction since he started eating food. I didn't want our luck to run out. I went into overdrive and moved all the snacks that contained peanuts or might have been cross contaminated onto the higher shelves of our pantry and fridge. I got him an allergy bracelet to wear and a t-shirt that alerted others of his allergy that he could wear at group gatherings. I educated all our friends and family about possible reaction foods with magnets for their fridges and pamphlets from a national food allergy group. I cut out all foods from his diet that were on the avoid lists because of cross contamination.

I kept my promise to that stranger in the bathroom in Chicago. When Alex's skin and then later his blood tests came back positive for peanut anaphylaxis, I took a positive hold of his allergy diagnosis and became his biggest and loudest protector. I made up pencil cases with his photo on them and all his medical information and *EpiPen* and medicines with instructions inside. This went in my bag and out the door with us every time we left home.

In my new understanding of what was at stake, I was going to be ever vigilant and very vocal about Alex's allergy until he was old enough to do it himself. I realized I couldn't be the only one keeping this growing, moving, grabbing body of his safe. I needed to train and trust others to watch his back until he could do so for himself. The best way to do that was to keep it front and center always.

Alex only knew of this in the way that a small, two-year-old child can, a simple matter of fact way. I told him that the cells in his body that were built to help him attack sickness were super sensitive hero cells, and for some reason, his cells were doing too good of a job. His body thought that peanuts were dangerous and attacked if he ate or touched them. I explained he would have to be careful of everything he put in his mouth and everything he touched to make sure it wasn't peanuts.

This broke my heart to make him aware of his limitations. But I had heard the doctor's directions. I thought we'd been lucky so far, especially since Alex was an extroverted walking and talking toddler. He was one of those kids that was always friendly to strangers and might touch or eat something unknown. I had to begin somewhere to get him to understand he couldn't eat peanuts, and he had to stop and ask before eating or touching a food item.

Alex took the peanut allergy debriefing just as if I'd told him the sky was blue. It was just a fact, another bit of information about the world from mom. Hearing him ask about peanuts for the first time both broke my heart and made me proud. "Peanuts in it?" his little voice asked loud and curious to the stranger offering him a sample at the grocery store. I knew he was safer already, and I felt better about my decision to tell him right from the beginning.

Over time, I started to understand the way food allergy safety works. I learned and felt and accepted this sobering effect: the more afraid, diligent, and alert you are, the better the odds. Constant fear and anxiety are the side effects to the lifelong prescription of food avoidance for a life-threatening allergen. Letting your guard down leads to increased risk of accidental ingestion, which means we were on high alert anytime food was a part of things. Food is everywhere. For a food allergy parent or sufferer, it is watched, dreaded, plotted, and checked daily, several times throughout the day, in fact, and even more so at any special events and outings. Food is laced into all parts of our lives and cultures. Fear and anxiety tag along and permeate every day and every interaction where food plays a role. This was not so much Alex's experience as it was mine. Remember to him allergic to peanuts at this point was like the sky is blue, just a given.

I became aware at all times how far we were from an emergency room. I became a person that no longer walked around carefree with just my keys and phone in my pocket and toddler on my hip. Instead I became a converted and devoted bag carrier. I carried my bag with the *EpiPen* in it always. I went from the concerned mom politely turning down the peanut butter cookie a stranger offered to a hyper vigilant vocal food allergy advocate advising others, even strangers, to not hand a kid food without checking with them or their guardian about food allergies first.

I became a label reading fiend. I was determined to cut all the minuscule peanut cross contamination out of his diet to help clear up his skin and give him comfort where I could. We treated the dust and grass allergies seriously as well and got dust mite covers for all beds. We put stuffed animals up, donated them, or washed them regularly. Our dear dogs became mostly outside dogs, or confined to the areas of the house without carpet.

We were a new food and environmental allergy team, making up for almost two years of complacency since the rattle incident, I felt committed to doing everything one hundred percent. Quickly, we got results from our diligence. Alex's eczema cleared up within a month or two of implementing avoidance of many things that he had previously eaten that were likely cross contaminated. My two-year-old finally had baby smooth skin on his forehead, arms, and legs that he had never had! This was visible, tangible proof that doing the hard work made Alex feel better in addition to being safer. Seeing this visible improvement in his skin was like a reward and made staying diligent tangible.

CHAPTER 3 - FIRST BITE

Emotionally preparing to prevent Accidental Ingestion

I settled in for the long, vigilant childhood. My eagle eyes were looking out for all the things I needed to remove from Alex's path. I focused on making him and the world around him as aware as I felt. For bursts of time, I felt in control, or at least in control of my anxiety. I believed that I could secure him in a peanut free existence, and that I had control over his safety. I rationalized that peanuts were easy to see in foods and easier to spot than some allergens. I got checklists from a national food allergy support group of all the foods to avoid if you were allergic to peanuts. I was armed with information, practiced on the *EpiPen* trainer, and knew that peanut butter could hide in chili and barbecue sauce. I was grateful that we had made it this far without Alex accidentally eating something. Now that I was aware, I was determined to ensure that nothing would get past me.

I would start to feel successful; after all, he hadn't tasted another toddler's food at a playgroup or park. I hadn't missed peanut listed as an ingredient on a label. But, then that bubble of control I thought I had would burst. As my mind went into the rabbit hole of all the things that hadn't happened, I would realize that I was staring down the hole of all the things that could still happen no matter how diligent and prepared we were. Then, the fear and anxiety would rush in, and the truth that when it came to food, control was an illusion.

There was no way I could control it all, no way to ensure 100% safety: over Alex's life so many people and places would touch and affect his food. That facet of food allergy was the bit that was hard to swallow and hard for me to feel at peace with. I had to be prepared and diligent and keep that fear and anxiety front and center informing every choice, but still I knew that no matter what I did, the worst could one day happen.

Physically preparing to prevent Accidental Ingestion

Shopping in the grocery store became a kind of research project. This was 2001, five years before the Food Allergen Labeling and Consumer Protection Act (FALCPA) that required all food labels in the United States to list top allergens. Without the added help of having allergens listed separately at the end of an ingredient list, it was tedious to read labels. I had never read food labels in my life! I was making sure the things I had been buying met my "may contain" and "cross contamination" standards.

Labels in those days could list obscure items like natural flavor or spices that could have allergens in them undisclosed. I remember calling manufacturers and requesting to know what items on the label meant and trying to get assurances they were peanut free. Some were unwilling to reveal their secret ingredients and those items didn't stay on my shopping list. Others, like Chi-Chi's salsa were extremely accommodating and revealed what those natural flavors were, solving the mystery for me on the spot. "So, that's why I love your salsa," I remember exclaiming to the customer service representative on the phone, "it has cilantro in it, and I love cilantro!"

On some calls, when I asked about the presence of peanuts I learned things that weren't on any label or my radar. For example, for one cookie I was told, "It doesn't have peanuts in it, but it is made on the same production line as cookies with peanut butter." So, off the list that cookie would go. And added to my head was a whole new level of anxiety. How many of the things that I thought were safe were made on contaminated production lines that I would never know about it? Why didn't food manufacturers have to disclose this information? I realized that homemade options for most baked and many processed foods were the only way to know for certain that peanuts weren't contaminating the food.

This forced label reading mania started an interest in what we were eating and what was in our food that has never gone away. If you can't pronounce it and don't even get to know what it is, why would you want to put it in your body? I am certain that label reading saved Alex from reactions over his life. A side benefit is that it likely gave our whole family a healthier eating experience. I dove right into the mindset of you are what you eat, so make it count.

The First Incident

Kurt and I made big strides in the year after Alex's diagnosis in educating ourselves and others and creating safe protocols. But, it wasn't all smooth sailing. There were some big mistakes. If we were a manufacturing facility with a sign counting the number of days since our last accident, we didn't rank very high. We only made it seven days. One glorious and successful week after filling Alex's *EpiPen* prescription, Alex ate peanut containing food and had a reaction. The allergist was correct in saying that a reaction was a *when* and not an *if.*

It happened right before Labor Day. I had stopped with Alex to visit Kurt at his long weekend shift at work. We were having lunch with daddy, something Alex loved to do. Kurt had stopped to eat and sit with us in the back of the retail store he worked in. We were two busy, tired parents, one of us five months pregnant, enjoying lunch with their toddler. We were still mesmerized daily at Alex, hearing all his cute accented words. Watching him explore the store and equipment and ask questions, we ate our lunch, us sitting, him roaming. As two tired parents trying to make a connection with each other in our busy days, this was a cobbled together lunch date.

I don't remember what we were talking about, but suddenly there was Alex in our faces, eyes wide and panicked. "Spicy, spicy, spicy!" he cried loudly but without the S pronounced fully at the beginning of each shouted word. His mouth was reddening around his lips; his eyes were red as well. The skin on the eyelids and underneath was red, and his nose was running, streaming.

Then I saw it, there on the floor, the dropped half of a peanut butter and jelly sandwich. Alex had reached up onto the edge of the counter in the back of the store where we were sitting and where Kurt had placed his lunch and grabbed Kurt's sandwich. Alex didn't know. It looked from a distance to him just like the sandwich I had made him sitting nearby on the chair we had fashioned into a table for him.

Quickly, we simultaneously assessed him and scanned our brains. We knew he had eaten peanut butter. We knew he was allergic. We were to assess his symptoms, and if needed, administer the *EpiPen* before it was too late and proceed to the emergency room.

I don't know that the scene was peaceful. It was our first epinephrine administration. I wish I'd had the foresight to be calm and not pass fear onto Alex, but my whole goal was stopping that reaction. He had taken a bite; I didn't know how much he had spit out when it tasted spicy and bad in his mouth and how much he had swallowed. With a reddening mouth and wide eyes, he began crying and grabbing at this throat saying his neck hurt. We held him, gave him water, calmed him, and listened. We both heard a difference in his breathing. He was wheezing and had heavier breathing sounds than normal.

I sat him in my lap in a chair and Kurt told him we were going to give him some medicine to stop the bad feelings. We told him that it might hurt for a second, but that we needed him to hold still. We explained that we had to use the medicine to help him and that it would make the spicy taste, hurting throat, and scary feelings stop quickly. I got the *EpiPen* out, and while holding Alex in my lap, Kurt firmly injected that needle we had so feared right into our baby's thigh. We then got in the car and headed to the emergency room nearby.

As we drove, I panicked every time Alex, strapped in his car seat, looked down or got excited and seemed bubbly and overstimulated. I kept thinking he was going to pass out or burst into song. We rolled the windows down and turned some music on. Epinephrine constricts blood vessels to prevent blood pressure from dropping, stimulates the heart, relaxes smooth muscles in the lungs to improve breathing, and reduces swelling caused by the histamine release. I didn't know it at the time, but epinephrine is a form of synthetic adrenaline. If I had known that, I wouldn't have been as worried as I was on the car ride.

I didn't know what epinephrine felt like in one's body, so I did not understand Alex's sudden up and down fluctuations. He was acting odd because it felt odd to be given a dose of adrenaline. Some of what the epinephrine was doing in his body I was reading as further reaction to the peanut. We made it to the ER; luckily, his reaction didn't escalate any further. His hives and respiratory reactions subsided. He got a follow-up standard steroid shot, and we sat with him for two hours while they monitored him in the ER.

This was a wakeup call. If I had not been scared enough by the education and training we had at the allergists a week ago, I sure was scared and aware now. I had seen a full anaphylactic reaction, and I had seen it stopped in its tracks by our quick actions and the epinephrine. I was humbled knowing that not even we could keep Alex safe from a reaction, and we were his parents. We just had to stay prepared. Each time we learned something new that could be a danger, or put Alex at risk, we needed to weigh that danger and decide what action to take.

Becoming even More Prepared

I decided after this incident that we could no longer have peanut products in our home for us to eat. Our need to eat those items did not outweigh the risk of Alex grabbing something we were eating like he had that day at lunch. Peanuts went completely off the menu in our home and off the family shopping list. I went home and threw away all the things that Kurt and I ate that still had peanuts in them. It felt horrible to have the reaction be our fault. I was determined to not have another accidental ingestion and reaction come from food we had bought and prepared.

Now that we knew better, we had to do better. We also decided that in addition to eliminating peanuts from our home, we would join Alex in peanut avoidance. The bubble of safety felt larger now that we knew it wasn't just Alex's ingestion we needed to worry about but also everything around him. The bubble and the boundaries of food avoidance we were setting felt more exact and easy to follow and likely to provide less anxiety and more safety. No peanut foods in our home meant no more chance of him accidentally grabbing something at home or from home. Kurt and I not eating peanut foods anymore meant that we could kiss Alex and hold him and not worry about causing a reaction, and we could feel free to share water bottles and drinks with him always without wondering what we had eaten earlier. He would not be alone in his avoidance, and we hoped we would never again be guilty of being the ones that inadvertently exposed him to his allergen.

Our awareness of how to handle Alex's allergy was an ongoing journey: every year, I realized at least one thing that needed to be handled differently. I remember seeing peanut butter residue in a jelly jar at a house and realizing suddenly that jelly at others' houses wasn't safe, and we needed to add that boundary. After he got a welt on his wrist while holding his sister's pet rat, I realized the rat food was cross contaminated. Through the years, I realized that birdseed, dog food, cat treats, and innumerable other items weren't safe from peanuts. Safe boundaries fluctuated when new information presented itself.

Coming across new things that were as dangerous as an actual peanut was like swimming in the Gulf of Mexico. At first it was the shark in the waters, the actual peanut or peanut butter in Alex's hand, that we knew to be dangerous and avoided. But knowing that shark attacks happen so rarely, we figured Alex would not be eating peanuts with the firm boundaries we had created. The reality of him eating a peanut, like a shark attack, seemed unlikely to happen.

We kept an eye out for those "shark's" fins sneaking into his diet and into his bubble, and when we saw one, we checked to see if it was a dangerous peanut "shark" or just a pod of harmless dolphins. Taking this ocean analogy a bit further, imagine on another visit to the beach, we learned while enjoying the waves, that yes, sharks are in the ocean, but they are not the only danger you have to watch out for. The waters are filled with jellyfish tentacles and manta ray barbs, and they are everywhere and can be just as dangerous as a shark attack. Then we were faced with the choice: to keep swimming and keep medicine and medical care on hand and know where the ER is just in case an accident happens or just stay out of the water completely. It's not just the sharks that you know about it's other things that are dangerous, too.

We never stopped helping Alex find ways to keep swimming fully in the waters of life. We did change his eating boundaries or food rules each time we learned of a new danger. But, we didn't keep Alex stuck in the sand unable to dip a toe in the water. In my analogy, the water is food contact out in the world—food is everywhere; it's a part of everything. We had to find ways to participate safely. Never getting in the ocean because there are sharks, never getting out in the world where the peanut containing food is, was not an option.

I know I grieved Alex having a food allergy diagnosis, but not consciously. Alex had his first full reaction biting Kurt's peanut butter and jelly sandwich in the weeks before the 9/11 attacks in New York. I was pregnant and my daughter was born months after in January of 2002. That fall and winter after Alex's diagnosis in August was a whirlwind. I fully embraced the control of food avoidance, and thought that I had it covered. I didn't mourn or lament the reality. So much around us in the climate of the country at the time seemed worse than having to avoid peanuts for life. We were alive, we were healthy, we had shelter and jobs and interests to follow and good to do in the world.

Looking back, internally I turned on some obsessive-compulsive disorder tendencies I had and I handled it with a calm, cool exterior. Inside I was a fearful, plotting, worrying mess. I ingrained peanut avoidance in every part of our lives. I gently and diplomatically put the fear for Alex's life in my dear family and friend's hands as well. I cringe at this, but I also put fear in Alex's hands. I cautioned him often and strongly to not eat food if he didn't know if it was safe or not. His two-year-old logic got it some but not totally. I wanted him to be afraid enough of eating something that his gregarious-do-anything personality would stop and pause before taking a bite. I had that recent peanut butter and jelly incident to remind him what it felt like to make a mistake eating something with peanuts in it and what the consequences and steps to take looked like.

I wanted him to have a healthy dose of fear and caution, but I also didn't want to ruin his zest for people or food or life. I didn't want him to develop an eating disorder or an irrational fear of touching things or food or other people. Wanting these two things, normal living and an abundance of caution, felt like an impossible tight rope to walk. If a situation occurred that I saw room for danger, I erred on the side of caution. I made Alex more afraid than an older child would have been so that he would stay safe until he could read and understand what was and wasn't safe to eat.

I know and see now that I was parenting him regarding situations with food based on fear and scarcity. That position was the opposite of all my other parenting strategies which were based on trust and love and an abundant view of the world. When it came to food, I coached Alex on how to survive instead of thrive. If it wasn't about food, I presented a worldview to him that was about thriving and abundance. These contradictions may have been confusing to him.

He didn't face survival or coping mechanisms with regards to any of his basic human needs such as food, shelter, love, and safety. He wasn't surviving anything drastic, so I don't mean to minimize actual abusive childhoods by claiming survival mode. But there was an undercurrent of survival that was front and center instead of the thriving childhood he might have had if it was unmarked by fear or the scarcity of activities and choices that food avoidance required.

It wasn't Alex with this fear and anxiety, it was me, and I was the mom he had. I was the one with the head of questions that was showing him the world. Unfortunately, peanuts acted as the running headline. When would he ingest it again? When it happened would he eat very much of it? Would it still taste spicy and would he exclaim it as loudly as he had before? Would the right adult be there to see what was happening in time? Would the *EpiPen* be nearby? Would Alex or someone else know to use the *EpiPen*? Would it save him again like it had in his first anaphylactic reaction? I do know this latent level of anxiety over 16 years affected my child.

CHAPTER 4 - TWICE BITTEN

Life Changes

It's hard to describe the reality of living in fear that your child will accidentally ingest food he shouldn't. Afraid of food and food events and food centered moments, that substance which all humans and cultures use to nourish, commune, connect and celebrate with, can be a lonely existence. I had to bury one connection to being human: knowing that food is life giving. We had to carry on living, watching out for innumerable things that most people never think about.

Five months after Alex's first anaphylactic reaction, my daughter was born, and I learned just how much I had been hovering around Alex both physically and mentally. Now that I had a baby in my arms, keeping Alex within sight and reach and safety became harder. On the playground, I had to play peanut spotter. I used to follow him around the playground seeing what things he was near, if anyone was eating peanut butter crackers on the top of the slide in the playhouse, if any kind child was sharing their candies. But, I could no longer do that easily with a baby in my arms. I became adept at using a baby carrier and a sling and my daughter didn't like to be put down, so she just flew around with me, like a second lieutenant on my peanut spying mission.

It was overwhelming to have this baby point out all I didn't know I was doing subconsciously to keep Alex safe. Overwhelming because I could see it immediately and yet I couldn't be or do more than my two arms, two legs, two eyes and two ears allowed. Seeing just how much I was watching out for him was another chance to reconfigure how to keep him safe. Alex's peanut secret service detail now had a baby in tow, so planning and reconnaissance skills had to be upgraded.

Integrating a new baby into a life of food avoidance with a toddler was not smooth sailing. It took years to get the extra eyes and extra caution to become second nature like they had been in the five months before Emma was born. The fog of having a new baby and training my brain to watch and care for more than one child took time especially with all the extra questions I had swirling around in my head that were specific to peanut avoidance. I was stressed and always preoccupied with an impending ingestion, stepping it out like a military maneuver in my head.

Despite the difficulties of an added child, at least home felt safe since we had removed everything that might have peanuts from within our four walls. It was the one space that I could totally relax and not worry. Everywhere else felt like I was going into battle. Deciding to go to the library story time could result in not coming home with Alex alive and intact. I replayed giving Alex his *EpiPen* in my head every time we left the house. I envisioned how I would hold Emma and Alex at the same time if I needed to administer the *EpiPen*.

I looked around at different venues to spot a safe place I could plop Emma down on the ground quickly to be able to help Alex. I found faces at the park that were complete strangers, but that I knew in a moment's heartbeat looked friendly enough that I could hand Emma to them in order to rush to Alex's side. No one at the park ever knew they were a part of this peanut storyline I was screenwriting in the background every day I was away from home. Again, this was my reality, not Alex's or anyone else's.

Mostly, it was an undercover and unknown, latent anxiety that I folded into the batter of being a new mom. I only saw it as abnormal when I didn't experience it with my other kids. Maybe I should have gotten counseling to frame it all differently in my subconscious, but I didn't, I just survived. This survival and constant state of anxiety affected my daughter. As I was constantly cloaked in anxiety, my baby and I did not have a calming environment. Google long term cortisol exposure; it's not a pretty picture. My daughter bore a sense of alertness and anxiety as a result of her body being "washed" in the stressed chemical makeup that was in my body while I was pregnant with her and breastfeeding her. She's an amazing, fully functioning teen today, but I know it affected her, and I regret that she and I didn't have a calm, stress free baby and mama hood together.

This didn't just affect my daughter; Alex's allergy affected our family. I don't know all the events or outings we weren't invited to after I became a militant food allergy advocate with friends and family. But I do know exclusion existed, not out of malice, but out of fear of hurting Alex or out of an inability by others to see how to do a specific thing with us safely. For some it was easier to not ask than creatively figure out a way, and I understood that, but it still hurt. I had two shining gemstones of friends in those toddler years that did everything under the sun to replicate a safe world for Alex and a safe space for me in our playgroups and in their homes.

Amy and Meg were the best friends a food allergy mom could dream of. They put away all peanut products. They took time in their tired days and mornings still in pajamas to wipe down their home's surfaces before we came over. They kept their children from touching things while eating peanut products if Alex was going to be around. They embraced it all: the scary, the hard choices, the truth of its importance. This was a big gift of love to us and to Alex. They told their kids about keeping Alex safe just like he had any other disability that deserved respect and consideration. I am forever grateful to them for that. They fully embraced some of the neurosis of a food allergy parent when they didn't have to, so Alex could feel and experience a normal hang out with friends while he was still so young, and it was hard to find spaces that felt that safe.

We survived year two in food allergy avoidance and with an added baby in the mix. A big part of me wanted to stay at home, at the safe understanding friends' houses, and in outside places only. I wanted to forego all group gatherings, especially those that involved food-like parties and meetings. The fact that I am introverted only added to that irrational wish of mine to exist at home until Alex was reading labels and demanding peanut free food on his own. However, I didn't become a homebody. I kept my highly extroverted and highly allergic child connecting out in the big scary world filled with peanuts.

Why did I do it? I wanted to defy this diagnosis. I wanted Alex to feel and be and experience *normal*. I didn't want the experience of motherhood for me and childhood for him and Emma to be taken by this nut. So, I did more to experience more. I volunteered to bring the cupcakes instead of the host getting them at Kroger, so I could make them and make sure they were safe and Alex could eat what everyone else was eating. This was 2002; there weren't any allergy friendly mixes in stores or allergy free bakeries, even in suburban Atlanta where we lived.

For a cake or dessert to be peanut safe, it had to be made by hand with a baby on my hip and a toddler at my feet. It was worth it to stay up late baking cupcakes to share in order to not make this allergy matter. I got weary of the sympathy and a bit irritated at the commentary others offered my way. The laments from others saying, "That must be so horrible to have a peanut allergy" were not kind. They told me that what I was doing was brave, that I was a superhero, and that they imagined they couldn't do it themselves. Well, of course you could do it if you had to, I would scream inside my head!

I know no one meant malice but rather meant to lift me up and congratulate me on keeping Alex safe. But I didn't want an award or sympathy. I wanted a shift in the culture of how we celebrate. I wanted other parents to get that humans and their safety mattered more than having a certain food at a gathering; that some foods and situations could be skipped or changed so an allergic kid didn't have to skip coming or leave a party early; I wanted food allergy safety to matter more than tradition about food. Food allergies being honored or treated as a protected status hadn't happened yet.

While I wished and hoped food allergies would be better understood in our culture, I don't regret choosing to allow Alex to brave the world, so that both he and I could feel normal, connected, and involved.

Second Bite

This desire to keep him connected did result in another incident. However, this time we kept him safe for a longer duration. We made it about eight months from the sandwich incident before peanuts hit again. It was at a La Leche League meeting (an international breastfeeding support group) in the spring of 2001 when his curious, playing, sharing hands reached into a bag of peanut butter cereal at that meeting and tasted away. The sweet of the cereal mixed with the spicy feeling and taste of the peanut confused Alex, and he didn't immediately come to me. This was a high-energy room of babies and moms and toddlers, probably more than thirty in all. It was the end of the meeting with the chaos of everyone talking one-on-one loudly over each other. Kids were circling the chairs and tables in games of chase and bodies were coming and going from the room.

In finishing my conversation and grabbing our bag to leave, I saw Alex across the room on the floor with some buddies. A friend was holding a plastic baggy of a crunchy sack. In my mind, it was like there was a venomous snake lying there on the carpet beside him. So many visuals became code red for me over the years for danger. Unknown unbranded carbohydrate snacks are one of those dangers. I made a beeline across the room for Alex and bent down to ask him to come with me. My intent was to just get him away from the unknown snack and head out the door.

When he raised his head to my voice, there on his mouth were the hives popping up. I panicked and asked him quickly but not calmly enough, "Did you eat something? What did you eat? Did you have some of your friend's cereal?" He shook his head no in anger because, obviously, my tone and my fear were confusing. He felt like he had done something wrong, so he said no to keep mom happy. Thankfully, his friend piped up loudly and said, "Yes, he did have some of my cereal. It's ok. I like to share; I told him he could have some." I smiled at his kind, honest friend and thanked him for telling me.

Turning away from the friend and Alex to plan, I handed Emma to a nearby mom, saying urgently, "Alex has likely eaten something with peanuts in it, and he's having a reaction, so please hold Emma. I have to help him." The snack sharing friend's mom overheard and gasped and confirmed, "Oh my god. I'm so sorry. Yes that's peanut cereal that we had in our bag from yesterday." I whisked Alex up telling him we needed to step outside the room and make sure he was ok. I had the forethought to know that I needed to get to a quieter room or hallway so that I could deal with what I was going to need to do. Nothing good would come of holding him down and administering his *EpiPen* while others stared in fear for him.

I already had his *EpiPen* in my diaper bag, and I carried him right into the next room, set him down in front of me, and considered his big brown eyes to assess and to connect. He had hives still, multiplying on his mouth and hands. I asked him to take a deep breath and reassured him that he hadn't done anything wrong, but that I needed to know how he felt: did his throat or neck feel funny, how did his stomach feel? In this brief exchange between us, he started to sneeze, consecutively several times. He told me his neck hurt (his words for throat) and that he had to go to the bathroom. I think he felt swelling and irritation in his esophagus or airway based on his neck hurting comment. I think his stomach felt icky based on his bathroom comment. I heard heavier breathing, but I have no idea if it was real or my perception. I saw those same concerned eyes that I had seen when he had screamed about the spicy sandwich. I remembered that I had practiced for this and that the *EpiPen* couldn't hurt him.

I picked Alex up and hugged him tight and told him I was going to be here with him and give him the shot to stop the reaction. He didn't want me to. With him crying, I held him in my lap and reminded him to be still so we could help his body. I felt horrible that I had to forcibly administer medicine, going against what I valued in teaching my child about consent and autonomy over his body.

The epinephrine and resulting trip to the ER were as successful this time as they were the time before. It was lifesaving, but each time it happened, I feared it eroded a bit of his autonomy in the world, a bit of his trust in me and the world as a safe place. This was a boy that wasn't made to hug family if he didn't want to. We had a family principle of raising him to respect others' space and his own space and that no meant no, and no was OK to say. Then here was this *EpiPen* injection whisking in to obliterate all of that. I feared that screwed with his little toddler head because it had sure screwed with mine already in the two times it had happened. How would I get our hearts out of this? We had a magic shot to heal his body from the deadly peanut. But, what could I do to heal any emotional damage?

An Accidental Lesson

A year and a half after the cereal incident, I was preparing to leave four-year-old Alex alone with a friend from Kurt's work. They were only going to be at our house where there were no peanuts around, but still I plotted the evening out. Being a visual person and very much in my head a lot of the time, I went to our laundry room to get out the *EpiPen* pouch and the *EpiPen* trainer and walk myself through the protocol again, a dress rehearsal of sorts. I was pantomiming what I was going to tell our friend about how the *EpiPen* worked: what you did, how you held it, how you removed the safety cap, where to inject, how to depress the device, how long to hold it in. In full rehearsal mode, I jabbed that trainer into my clothed thigh only to realize that I wasn't holding the trainer but rather the actual *EpiPen*! I had accidentally injected myself with epinephrine.

Within moments the adrenaline coursed through my body, and I was racing inside and this was only the *EpiPen* Jr. dose for children. With my heart beating, breathing quickening, and every cell of my body feeling jazzed, I began to understand exactly how my little guy had felt the two times we had treated him. Well...I knew how his body felt after the reaction; I could never know what it felt like to feel the fear, struggling to breathe and throat tightening from eating an allergen. However, at least I knew how he felt post injection, and this helped me talk him through future injections. I, jokingly, highly recommend that if you ever accidentally inject yourself with epinephrine, it's worth it! Don't feel stupid or careless, embrace the mistake for the insider knowledge it gives you. It got me completely over the fear of administering because I felt it, needle and all. It was not as big of a deal as the anticipation or idea of it in my head. It also gave me first person data for those later harder conversations Alex and I would have about him learning to self-administer.

CHAPTER 5 - FIRST AND LAST SCHOOL

Preventing exposure became my number one parenting priority. I felt comfortable with the people whom I had educated and now trusted to handle Alex's allergy, so I was not as willing to venture out of that safe bubble. I had lists of foods memorized that might contain peanuts. I watched all the contamination websites weekly to see if a random production flaw had contaminated a previously safe food item. While it was a lot of effort, this diligence in watching labels led to not eating as much processed food.

By default, in needing to read labels, I fell into a parenting group of "natural" families in the Atlanta suburbs. We had normal weekends of visiting the DeKalb Farmers Market, and I spent time throughout the week after making homemade meals. Eating whole foods and "natural" family living became the framework for decision making and finding like-minded friends. My new group of friends discussed education and where to send their kids before their child could even crawl.

Georgia adopted public Pre-K programs, so at the age of four, a child could enroll in the public-school system for full day Pre-K programs. Many took education seriously, and it felt competitive: What district schools had the best teachers? What private schools or church schools had better outcomes? What advantages were there to a natural learning approach like Montessori or Waldorf to help your child succeed as a member of society? What advantages did preschool give a child? Was it more beneficial to have a parent stay at home as long as possible with young children and let them play rather than attend school at such a young age? These were all important questions I heard murmured around me.

When Alex turned four in the fall of 2003, I started looking for a program for him to begin his school journey. We wanted the best for him and knew he would enjoy the social aspects of school. Also, with Emma around, I felt I needed Alex off learning with others for the day so I could be a mom to Emma, too. The first school I visited for Alex was the new elementary school within two miles of our home. This school had been built in the past five years and yet already had portable temporary school classrooms dotting the school grounds.

I entered the school excited and ready to get Alex interested. My mom was an amazing kindergarten teacher for 25 years, so I had a lot of expectations about Alex's first school experience. We toured at the open house, and I was impressed and astounded at the size of the school. It was a different world than the one class per grade elementary school I had gone to as a kid in a smaller city. This elementary school had six or more pre-k classrooms alone. It was a lot to digest. It was hard to imagine Alex staying safe throughout the day with his peanut allergy without our eyes watching out for him.

After the initial tour, I went back via appointment to talk to the office staff, the nurse, and the principal about how they integrated food allergy safety into the classrooms and overall school. Despite being armed with information to share from national allergy support groups and a reasonable set of safety protocols, the school administration was not able to meet any of the needs that Alex had to be safe. Either due to the size of the school or where we were on the timeline of food allergy awareness, there wasn't an adequate understanding or protocols in place to handle food allergies safely in this school. This was a deal breaker for me.

To the best of my knowledge, this was before the widespread advent of 504 plans, individual health plans, or food allergy action plans that are honored in most school systems in the United States today. I was requesting concessions that weren't mainstream yet to keep Alex safe. The school was unable to meet them, and I didn't take it any farther than that meeting. I didn't have the energy or knowledge to know I could demand protections.

For example, they did not have separate nut safe tables for kids to eat at in the school. They did not allow *EpiPens* to be in Alex's bag or accessible to his teacher in the classroom he would be in. All *EpiPens*, treated like a medicine dispensed at a certain time, would be under lock and key with only two people on the premises having access to the locked cabinet, the nurse and the principal. The administrators weren't rude; they just didn't have the knowledge that I had of what it meant to keep Alex safe.

The *EpiPen* being that far away time-wise wasn't safe. The lack of a safe table to eat lunch was an accident waiting to happen. The sheer number of children in the school amplified every risk and fear I had for Alex's safety. I could not see putting Alex in a dangerous situation just to start him on a school path, so I went searching for learning options elsewhere.

Next I considered private and church preschool programs and Montessori schools. I thought that they would be more individualized and accommodating of Alex's food allergy needs. I figured he could go to a private school setting until he was older, and then he would better understand the role he played in keeping himself safe, and we could transfer him to a public school. In the back of my head, I was also still holding out hope that instead of Alex's allergy being lifelong, he would be one of the 20% of peanut allergic kids that outgrow their allergy by age eight or ten. So, I just needed to plan for him at four and five years old when he couldn't keep himself safe.

I was wrong about the private or church preschools near us being more accommodating. These preschools also had busy full, crowded programs and no protocols in place to provide a safe learning environment. They seemed even more casual and unaccustomed to addressing medical issues like food allergy than the public school had been.

Food was a part of each day, twice a day, and even sometimes in the crafts. When I asked about possible exposure to peanut products throughout the year at special activities like holidays, one teacher said that it wouldn't be a problem. She explained that if they were doing the fall craft of making peanut butter and birdseed covered pinecones, she could just help Alex do something else while the rest of the class did the project. Hearing this, I realized the education gap on peanut allergy was wide, and it seemed unsurmountable. This teacher didn't understand the infeasibility and danger of having a peanut allergic child in a room with other children smearing peanut butter on pinecones and desks and doorknobs! I got out of that place quickly, nearly having hives myself.

I visited a Montessori school that had rave reviews by other parents. On the tour, I found they had a station that contained peanuts. In order to practice "practical life" skills, they had a food area for children to use to prepare their own snack. This station had juice and water to pour in tiny pitchers as well as cheese and apples to practice cutting and peanut butter to spread on crackers. When I asked if the room Alex was assigned to could be kept free of peanut butter, I didn't get a resounding yes.

They suggested that Alex not use the peanut butter and that it might help him learn to avoid it out in the real world by avoiding it in the classroom. They had greater confidence in my 3.5-year-old than I did. They assured me that the other kids always ate their snack on the work area's trays so other surfaces in the room would remain contact safe for Alex. I rolled my eyes internally, but resigned myself that this otherwise amazing, serene, learning environment was also not going to work for us. I could have insisted for accommodation and educated them further, but honestly once I heard their suggestion, I lost all trust in leaving Alex alone there as well.

Next I found another Montessori school to explore. I had liked the principles I was exposed to at the first Montessori I toured. This second place ended up being a dream come true. It was owned and operated by another allergy mom that had a peanut allergic child herself! How lucky could we get? They had a whole classroom in their school that was designated the "nut free" room and the teachers in that room were trained in food allergy safety and reaction procedures. The *EpiPen* could be kept in the room with the teacher and assistant and owner all having access. Not surprisingly, we enrolled him that winter.

Alex adjusted well for about five months before we hit another roadblock. Montessori has a tradition when it's a child's birthday called the Celebration of Life. The birthday child gets to invite his or her family in to share in the celebration and gets to bring in a healthy treat for sharing with the class. In the Celebration of Life, there is a setup depicting the months of the year and the sun is represented by a candle in the center. The birthday child walks around this "sun" for each year of their life hearing stories about themselves and sharing pictures. At the end, there is a song and then it is treat time for the class if the family brought treats. After about four months of attending, Alex's class had a child celebrating a birthday that had chosen to have his family join and bring a birthday treat to share.

The bump in the road was this birthday treat the family brought for the class. I didn't know the celebration was happening that day when I dropped Alex off or I would have talked to him about it, warned him, and planned with his teacher. After the celebration of life that day, the birthday child's parent went around the room handing out muffins, and when they got to Alex, they offered him a muffin. Alex said no because his little four-year-old brain was learning to say no to food that wasn't his own safe food. The visiting family member didn't know anything about Alex's allergy, and the teacher wasn't aware there was something happening at Alex's table. The parent, instead of hearing Alex's no, gave him a muffin anyway, putting it in his hand. In fear, Alex lost control and had a crying, terrified meltdown in the room. I was called to pick him up. I rushed to the school confused, but before I left, we had figured out through conversation with Alex and the teacher what had happened.

The safe feeling Montessori room was never the same for Alex after that. For a month afterwards, he cried and refused to go every morning and was inconsolable at the door at drop-off time. After trying all ways of easing him back into it, I was finally exhausted and frazzled, especially since I had my one year old with me. It seemed silly to keep forcing him to try and go and stay without me there. He did not feel safe and helping him feel safe took precedence.

I hated that he was afraid to go to Montessori because of a food incident. I didn't know how to undo the fear at that level and at his age. It is something we have talked about his whole life, undoing the fear of an incident and starting over. That conversation began here at Montessori with this muffin incident, but we had many further conversations on how to have a healthy dose of food caution without fear and anxiety. I think he's come out of the other end as unscathed as he can be with needing to be cautious and fearful of food. We brought him back home that May when it was clear this wasn't a learning option anymore.

And thus began my exploration of homeschooling. Homeschooling was certainly on the extreme end of the spectrum, in my opinion, regarding protecting Alex. It was a path that I tried to avoid but given the public-school options and the safest private school feeling unsafe to him, there wasn't anywhere else to turn. I researched homeschooling methods, found one that fit my personality and ideals and Alex's energy and learning style, and gave it a go.

In deciding to homeschool, I was unaware of all the changes the school system made over the next decade in regards to food allergies. As such, I didn't experience handling food allergies in a private or public school system. I have filled out Food Allergy Action Plans for numerous occasions and advocated for my son's allergy as a medical condition at many events, for team sports, field trips and camps, but that is the extent of my knowledge. I've never had to advocate for my child or fill out a 504 plan for my child's food allergy in a school system.

I am grateful for the dedicated parents that challenged many school's lack of willingness to accommodate food allergies in the first decade of the 2000s when safety was low. They won more protections and safety for food allergic kids nationwide.

Growing up, I peripherally knew people that homeschooled. My mom's friend homeschooled her kids. We visited occasionally when my mom was there for a meeting. This family's house was wild and full of abandon unlike the organized canvas at my home. Remember my home was that of an orderly elementary school teacher! Their house had experiments roaming on every surface.

The oldest son had a huge boa constrictor living in a cage that he fed live rats to. There was chaos living with a kind of freedom and certainty that was magnetic to me as a child. They had the best climbing tree and forts in the backyard that I explored with their daughter. I learned to ride a bike at this house in their driveway and on their street. These were the most intriguing homeschoolers I knew growing up. Learning in this environment looked and felt normal and carefree. It was as if they hadn't chosen to homeschool for safety or protection from ideas but rather to full on embrace the beautiful mess that is human exploration.

Most other homeschoolers I was exposed to as a child were more structured. They had taken their kids out of school for reasons that were about sheltering and protecting them from culture and ideas. For most, religion was at the heart of their family decision to homeschool. Their kids were always well dressed, prepared, and had a yes and no ma'am in every sentence. It was a rigidity that alarmed me; I couldn't see myself in that kind of a teacher role. I didn't want to police my kids all day. How could I be their teacher and not wear that authoritarian hat?

I had some preconceived notions of what homeschooling was and what it looked like. I came into my adult years with pretty set expectations and judgements about what was a valid and valued educational path, and that certainly didn't include homeschooling. It included learning inside the system that was set up and then going on to college.

Even as I started homeschooling Alex, it was a big blow to my dreams for him. I couldn't even shepherd him comfortably through private Montessori schools to get him to the education system I saw and dreamed of him participating in. I grieved at it not working out as I'd planned. It was an internal struggle as to what to do. Enroll him again and risk ingestion or contact or his escalating anxiety, or take the path I had judgements about and homeschool him?

We moved soon after, when Alex was five, to a different state and district with smaller schools. I wanted to keep the option of attending school open to Alex as he got older and getting out of the big city was a part of that. Our intuition and time eventually made the final decision for us. He was a young five-year-old kid. As I researched more on learning and different approaches and became more comfortable with the idea of homeschooling, I came to the decision that enrolling him in the best school program was not a life or death decision for his future. It was more important for him to be a child as much as possible and play and learn without anxiety and fear. This meant embracing homeschooling until circumstances changed for him, for the school systems, or for his allergy.

I did a complete 180 degree turn on my erroneous view of homeschooling. Our homeschooling ended up looking different than the stereotypical view of homeschooling I had from childhood that I was afraid of. It turned out, as I got into the homeschooling community, that even in Alabama, where we now lived, my preconceptions were wrong.

It was not only families desiring to bring their faith into their learning that kept their kids at home to learn. Online groups connected me to families near and far choosing to learn outside of the school system not for religious reasons, not for food allergy or other medical reasons but because, for their kids, learning happened better at home. School had changed since I was a kid, and there was more testing and performing that had overtaken the wonder and curiosity. Year by year our reasons for homeschooling became less and less about keeping Alex safe from peanuts and more and more about keeping us sane and happy life learners.

By the time the school culture regarding food allergies changed as it did over the next few years, I no longer wanted Alex to attend school. We had built a network of homeschooling friends and groups and an enjoyable pace of learning at home that fulfilled our needs. I didn't realize it, but I wasn't searching for a school anymore. We had created our own version of that rich, chaotic learning system that I had witnessed at my mom's friend's house growing up. It was messy, our learning was rarely linear, and it was not defined by subjects but rather by interests or projects. Most days, it was a path of learning full of wonder and freedom. Our homeschooling style, if given a label, migrated from Montessori to eclectic, to project or unit based, to whole life learning, to unschooling. It was an unfolding through the years of what worked best for each child.

Since we didn't have food freedom, I quested for freedom everywhere else I could grasp it, including how to home educate. I wanted abundance instead of scarcity everywhere I could place it; thus, my homeschooling took paths that excitedly fired all my searching for freedom landing me at unschooling.

This definition of unschooling by Kelly Lovejoy is what it means to me: "If you knew you only had a year more with that child, what would you expose him to? Where would you go? What would you eat? What would you watch? What would you do? If you had only ONE year—and then it was all over, what would you do? Four seasons. Twelve months. 365 days. Do that THIS year. And the next. That's how unschooling works. By living life as if it were an adventure. As if you only had a limited amount of time with that child. Because that's the way it IS."

I wholeheartedly believe in the tenets of learning using unschooling principles. While I do identify as an unschooler, the key was this style allowed me to say YES to many things when the peanut stood there threatening so much NO in Alex's childhood.

Alex was thriving at home and protected from both peanuts and anxiety. Feeling safe and settled, his brain and body were free to learn and be. It seems odd to do a non-normative thing, like homeschooling, and to feel normal, but that is what I think happened. I think the best way for Alex to have the normalcy of childhood with regards to being able to be a carefree child with others and in group settings was to bring him home.

Instead of putting him in those large group spots filled with unknowns and anxiety for him and for me, I worked hard to either bring the world to us or bring him to the world safely in other ways in those early years. I wanted to heal the anxiety he had taken on with that muffin. Instead of homeschool teacher, I mentally assigned myself the role of tour guide. As tour guide, I filled days and weeks with exposure to people of all ages and group sizes as we learned from home.

Homeschooling is not something that I would have considered without the initial push of having a peanut allergic child. It quickly went from last resort in my brain to first choice after about two years of living it daily. Learning at home and from life; on the road while traveling; on nearby adventures and field trips; and wherever Alex's, and later our other kids', interests took them ended up being the brightest silver lining in this peanut allergy cloud. My friend, Esther, has a beautiful word and definition for this style of learning: she called it Roamschooling when I met her. She explains it as *"Roamschooling is to roam: roman, from Old English ramian "act of wandering about"* and *school: Old English scol, from Latin schola, from Greek skhole 'leisure, spare time'." (Crawford, 2005).*

I am grateful that Alex's peanut allergy gave me pause when it came to education. It was a gift to have him and then later our other kids learning at home.

At the tail end of the childhood learning journey, my fears of homeschooling seemed silly. Alex is a junior now, and he has all the same college and other opportunities in front of him, if he chooses to take them, that he would have had he gone to school. I like to think that for him, keeping him home saved him anxiety in those formative years. It has been the greatest gig of my life so far to have chosen and been fortunate enough to be home full time and working from home with my kids while they grow and learn. To be their tour guide and not just their Uber ride has been a big food allergy bonus.

CHAPTER 6 - THIRD BITE

We improved our protection skills considerably from the time Alex was 2.5 until he turned 8. From 2002 to 2007, we had a solid five and a half years without an accidental ingestion. The counter, the imaginary one on the factory floor of my head measuring days passed since last accident, was showing over 2,000 days of safety success. This felt like a record-breaking number. After having two reactions in less than two years at the beginning, I was feeling proud and good about this gap.

I also knew that success carried the stress of diligence and that wore on me no matter the outcome. Constant and frequent raised cortisol levels leave their mark on bodies and minds. So despite reaching 2,000 days of accident free living, I have these marks, my battle scars.

This five-year span made me comfortable with the control. It became second nature, like a second skin I wore unaware. Honestly, I was in marathon mode. I still thought I could out distance run this nut. I didn't tell Alex of my hope that he would outgrow his peanut allergy. When others around him asked, I offered that it was unlikely. I didn't want him to become complacent or hopeful and have his hopes crushed.

We had been so thorough and exact for over five years, and I dreamed Alex would outgrow his allergy. He could be in that 20% statistic. He was exceptional. If anyone could be in that statistic, it was my kid! I was hopeful, and honestly, I believed it could happen. I was also naïve thinking my diligence in keeping him clear of peanuts would have a positive effect on his ability to outgrow his allergy. But, onward to the finish line, I ran towards that 8-year mark. I expected he would show lower allergy levels when the time for blood tests came.

Perhaps, creating this expectation is part of what gave me the energy to keep going diligently for five years. It was an exhausting task to stay food safe. I had done mind tricks and given myself an end goal: I just had to make it to eight or nine years, and then his blood work would show he no longer had the allergy. Then we could proceed through the rest of Alex's childhood without the constant diligence and the fear of losing him to a bite caused by a reaction that didn't get treated in time.

Alex was no longer a toddler. He had just turned 8. He had two younger siblings, an active homeschool group of friends, and outings and play dates in our neighborhood. He had played soccer and practiced Tae Kwon Do; gone on vacations with family and friends, both with us and without us; traveled on planes successfully; participated in day camps. As more people entered the scene with food allergies, it became more common and commonplace to know others with an allergy. There were accommodations and exceptions built into activities to account for food safety.

Alex and I were in a different place five years out from the last time he ate a peanut out of his friend's cereal bag. We were allergy veterans. Alex didn't specifically remember the reaction he had at two and a half. Life avoiding peanuts was just normal and second nature for him.

It was a normal Halloween with our eight-year-old, six-year-old, and two-year-old. Alex was a spider, Emma was a butterfly, and Owen was a precious gum ball machine. We have always loved Halloween even though it is a notoriously difficult holiday for food allergy. The dressing up, the creativity, the crisp time of year moving into darkness and reflection.

We had a system for enjoying Halloween that kept Alex safe and participating. He would trick or treat with all the other kids in the neighborhood, but then mom and dad went through all the candy afterwards and pulled out the unsafe ones, and he got to replace them with his own bags of candy that were nut safe. At each doorway, he chose or asked for something that was peanut free. I usually ordered him some nut-free chocolates online from a vendor that served the allergy community. We then donated the unsafe candy to the local hospitals or businesses the day after Halloween. The other kids in our family did this as well. This way, in the end, there was no peanut candy in the house.

Halloween of 2007 happened. The candy was filtered, and we went back to a completely safe and peanut free home. In a great show of love and inclusion, Alex's friends always agreed not to eat their peanut candy while walking around trick or treating with him. He had some real compassionate heroes at his side, great friends. This kept contact risk at a minimum for Alex. All of this is what made Halloween as normal as possible. Our kids then consumed their bags of Halloween candy in the following weeks. They tended to savor it instead of consume it all at once.

That year instead of buckets or pillowcases or plastic pumpkins, the kids each had a recycled gift bag that they used for candy collection. These bags were left over from Alex's birthday earlier in the month. At the end of the night, I dumped Alex's candy bag out on the counter and sorted all the safe items from the non-safe items. There weren't many unsafe things, a random Mary Jane candy that had snuck in. Some cross contaminated mini Hershey bars in a variety of flavors, some unknown chocolates. If you aren't familiar with Mary Jane candies, they are made of peanut butter or crushed peanuts and molasses or perhaps corn syrup today. They have been around since 1914 when they were first sold as penny candies in dime stores. Being a vintage candy, they have retained their vintage shape and wrapper. They are a rectangle shape about 50% smaller than a domino and the chewy candy is wrapped in yellow wax paper with one red stripe and a small girl named Mary Jane (supposedly the founder's aunt) pictured.

Then like always, there was a double check. Kurt would do the same thing I had. He dumped all the candy out and went through it piece by piece to make sure I hadn't missed anything. Alex was a part of this process. He was trying to learn to read the complex labels on foods. We were trying to make him a part of everything that we could. Individually packed candy often doesn't have labels, so there wasn't a lot he could learn from this process, but he was there soaking up information. After the double check was complete, the candy bag went to Alex to consume as he wished. I relaxed a little, another Halloween was completed successfully. We were in the clear, or so I thought.

One night later that next week, I was in the kitchen cooking dinner. Alex was deeply engaged in learning and enjoying a new game on the computer that was set up in the den in view of our kitchen. At one point, he zoomed through the kitchen and threw something in the trash. I wasn't aware of this at the time but my subconscious was.

Soon after that, he came to me and said that his throat hurt. I was surprised and asked him how long it had been hurting. He told me that it just started hurting. I asked more questions, probing him if it started in the morning or the afternoon. He replied no to all my questions and told me that it had started hurting just now while he was playing the computer. I offered to make him some hot tea and give him some throat spray if he wanted. He said yes to the tea and declined the throat spray.

Before he went back to the computer, he asked if I would make him a snack. I asked if he could wait a few minutes, explaining that dinner was almost ready. He told me he could, but he needed to get this bad taste out of his mouth first. My ears perked up. At this point my attention to dinner stopped and went right onto Alex and assessing him. Apparently, for me, "bad taste" was a code red word.

"What bad taste?" I calmly asked him. He then shared the truth he didn't know he was hiding, "Well, mom, one of my candies was rotten; it tasted bad so I want that taste out of my mouth." By now all my alarm bells were going off in surround sound.

"What candy did you eat? Where is it? Can you show me the wrapper? I am worried that maybe you ate something with peanuts in it." I lobbed all those questions and information at him in seconds. The look of doom washed over him instantly, and he started to cry, afraid of what he could likely only remember in his subconscious and what he had been told over the years. The last time he had a reaction he was 2.5 years old. His 8-year-old self couldn't remember that other than the feeling of it.

"I spit it out in the trash can," he told me through his tears. I remembered then being aware of him whisking through the kitchen recently and the noise of the trash can opening. I quickly opened the trash can and saw a brown, unrecognizable caramel looking blob on the top of the trash. I was confused, I didn't recognize this candy or know of a caramel that was unsafe that was in his candy bag. "Where is the wrapper?" I quizzed him.

I had two devils on my shoulders talking in my ears. One, a rational voice, said this wasn't a reaction because it was different than before, he has no hives, he hadn't said it was spicy, and maybe he just had a sore throat coming on as it was that time of year; I didn't need to over react. The other devil screamed at me: listen to your intuition; remember it can't hurt him to inject; you should just grab the *EpiPen* and do it and model for Alex not to hesitate. I wanted to find a more angelic and balanced voice to speak calmly to both the logic and the intuition and help Alex and me get to a sound action plan.

Alex told me he didn't know where the wrapper was. I needed to know if we could find the wrapper and discerned we had a minute to look since there were no symptoms beyond his sore throat. I went to the candy bag and checked all the wrappers. I scoured the floor in his room. I headed next to the computer desk and there on the desk was a Mary Jane wrapper. The wrapper stood out to my trained peanut spotting eyes.

The mystery was solved, and it wasn't good news. I got Alex right in front of me, explained the reality and told him we needed to assess what was happening in his body and how much if any he had ingested. I explained that he hadn't done anything wrong, and I had no idea why there was an unsafe candy in his candy bag. I apologized for my part in it because his dad and I had checked the candy in his bag twice.

His throat was still hurting; he said it felt worse. He told me his stomach was hurting as well. I had him lie down on my bed and assessed his breathing which was heavier and more audible than normal, not a full wheeze, but labored. I was perplexed at the lack of hives, but I also knew that not every reaction was the same and Alex had three body systems reacting: throat swelling, respiratory and gastrointestinal. I knew he needed to have his *EpiPen* and proceed to the ER.

I asked Alex before I went any further if he wanted to give himself his *EpiPen* or if he wanted me to. He replied he didn't want the *EpiPen* at all. I explained that wasn't an option as he had a reaction happening, and we needed to stop it to keep his body working. I told him he was too precious to me to waste any time stopping the reaction. I reassured him that his fear over the few seconds of the needle was exactly what he had to get over to be able to one day inject himself.

I told him what it would feel like because I knew from my accidental injection. I told him I would do it for him quick, but I needed him to sit still on my lap. I prepared to administer his *EpiPen* while he sat still on my lap, but protested with, "No, no, no, I don't like it." I encouraged him to look away. He was so brave through this moment. He knew it had to happen, but he also wanted the alternate reality to exist that it didn't have to happen.

We did it, crying together, and in seconds it was over. Again, I am haunted by having to do what felt like force even though I wasn't holding him down. I felt like I had stripped him again of his autonomy and trust in me. But, I didn't see any way around it. We went to the emergency room, and the reaction subsided. In this instance, the hives came later in the ER after we were there.

I consider this third bite a good accident. It might seem odd to say this. I know parents of food allergic children, myself included, find pride or peace or reassurance of safety in going through childhood or for long times without having an ingestion. It seems best to not have to use the *EpiPen* and go to the ER for a reaction. In childhood, the years from two and a half to eight are a lifetime developmentally both physically and emotionally. Since this happened at age eight, I now knew that Alex was fully aware of his peanut allergy. He didn't remember the other two times he had a reaction and *EpiPen* when he was young any more than he remembered a busted chin at two or his round of vaccinations as a toddler.

Gained Confidence

I thought any future reactions would feel the same as it had at age two: hives on his mouth, spicy taste that he would be able to relate to what he had eaten. But I was wrong. And so, for that awareness alone, I was grateful this had happened as I reflected on it. It was his respiratory and gastrointestinal system reacting primarily this time. He didn't develop hives until later that night, perhaps as the allergen digested? Also, the spicy taste that we had always talked about with him wasn't what his eight-year-old brain called spicy anymore. He could talk about it with me and tag it in his memory as tingly on his tongue. Since the Mary Jane was a candy laced with sugar, it was a tricky feeling on the tongue; he didn't consider at the time he ate it that it was an ingestion of peanut. We got to talk about how the allergen could be hidden and not seem suspect at first.

His body and brain now knew what it felt like to accidentally ingest. I had confidence that I hadn't known I was missing. The next time it happened if I wasn't there, he would be more likely to recognize it and get himself safely cared for. Alex didn't administer the *EpiPen* this time, but we had conversations about him doing it the next time it happened. We gave words and plans to the hurdle he would have to get over in that moment to be able to do it himself. Our role plays with the epinephrine "trainer" now had a real-life scenario to give him relevance.

Despite this mistake that could have turned tragic, he now had an education and understanding of keeping himself safe that I doubt I could have imparted to him otherwise. He also got a step closer to conquering the fear he had about the needle of the injector. After it was over, he realized that the idea of the needle was actually worse than the injection itself.

I let go of a little bit of the fear I had with how he would handle a reaction without me around. I didn't even realize I was holding that inside me. While that fear was gone, I held onto guilt for a few days for failing to spot the candy and allowing him to have a reaction on my watch again. Then I let that guilt go like the old balloon it was, useless and not helpful to moving forward.

Turning on the mind tricks again, I found a way to forgive myself and turn the moment into some grace. I focused instead on finding all the things to tag onto this moment that would benefit Alex handling his allergy in the future. In my opinion, this reaction was my worst mistake to date. I decided to sweeten that sour lemon of a thought into lemonade. This had created more safety for Alex down the road.

After we got home from the ER, we dealt with Alex staying up late and riding out the energy the steroid shot gave his eight-year-old body. During that time, I decided I had to figure out how we had missed that Mary Jane candy. The extreme mom in me wanted to throw the whole candy bag away and ban candy eating and Halloween for life. The rational mom in me knew there was a way to learn from this and to walk in empowerment to keep fear at bay.

I got his candy bag out again. When I went to dump it on the counter, I realized that the cardboard piece that sits in the bottom of most gift bags was askew inside the bag. In rummaging with my hand, I saw that candy could have been stuck or lodged under the folded seams at the bottom of the bag covered by that cardboard piece. This must have been where that Mary Jane hid for that week. I know both Kurt and I double checked the candy, and we couldn't have both missed it if it were visible.

I performed the same gift bag bottom dissection on the other kids' bags in case they had a straggler peanut candy in their bag to get it out of the house as well. They didn't have any hiding candy in their bags and life moved on into the holidays. Alex's third bite reaction had happened. He had survived and was better informed than before. Alex had an idea of what being aware and on high alert meant. His mind had grown overnight because he knew more about and held more responsibility for his allergy.

CHAPTER 7 - LAST CHANCE TO OUTGROW

Second Test

It was finally time to get a blood test again and see what Alex's levels were doing. We journeyed to the allergist we used in an adjacent city, underwent the blood draw, and awaited the results. For Alex, I don't think there was an expectation of any news or change; it was just a blood draw and a test related to his allergy. Since I hadn't shared the possibility with him or the statistics about some kids outgrowing allergies, he lived like peanut avoidance was forever. I wanted him completely focused on avoiding, not getting confused with the idea that one random day in the future peanuts might be safer than they were now. I also didn't want him to be disappointed. He was at peace with his allergy status as it was all he'd ever known.

The blood results came back high. The research indicated that with these lab results, Alex would not outgrow his allergy. This news was a blow to me. I went through another step of grief and accepted with finality that his peanut allergy, its severity, and life complexity were here to stay. It wasn't going away. It was no longer a control and protect race we could celebrate finishing once we reached mile marker eight, nine, or ten. It didn't matter how well we had done avoiding peanuts, food allergy life wasn't leaving.

In some ways finally knowing that his peanut allergy was here to stay was freeing. I stopped holding my breath a little bit after this news. I focused on a lot of the realities of the prior eight years and the realities that were stark and unchangeable for Alex. And as I did so, I finally got angry. And I mean scary, crying, sobbing angry, both alone and with Kurt.

Then I wiped my tears away and put that anger to work. I got down to the serious business of preparing my little guy to be on his own in the world with this as his truth. He had to learn to say all the things to waiters and strangers that I did. He had to learn to read labels himself. He had to be his advocate because I had to know he could do it one day when we weren't there anymore. He had to be able to give himself his epinephrine.

There were tears in the years after this test took away any hope of Alex outgrowing his allergy. Alex didn't want to talk about the handling of his peanut allergy as much as I wanted him to talk about it with me. As he wasn't used to hearing all the internal dialogue I had about an event regarding his allergy spoken out loud, it was unsettling. It was probably embarrassing at times even alone with just me. It was a big weight for me to be pulling out of my sleeve and asking him to carry.

This shift was gradual over several years, but intentional. I wanted to have a teenager who could go off to camp or for a week at a time anywhere for that matter and be as safe with himself as a peanut protector as he was with me. I insisted that he had to carry his own epinephrine; it could no longer be stored in my bag but rather had to be on his body or in his bag. This was hard for him because he didn't like to carry a bag like my daughter did. The *EpiPen* 2-pack was bulky, so you couldn't fit it in your pocket. When the *Auvi-Q* brand epinephrine injector finally came to market for a brief time before it was recalled, Alex was ecstatic. It fits easily in a boy's pocket. I'm glad to hear it's coming back to market in 2017.

I asked Alex to ask the questions at restaurants and ask for the manager when they weren't answered well enough by the server. I was still there to help but beside him not in front of him. It felt like tough love that I wasn't interested in dealing out, but it was all in the name of life skills he needed to survive with his food allergy. If I could see him learn it and do it while I watched and acted as the voice on his shoulder, then I could better trust he would do it once he was alone. This was another step as he got older in my doing all I could to keep him safe.

Not only did we begin teaching Alex to be his own self-advocate, but we enlisted his siblings as well. We were shifting the sole ownership of protecting Alex from off our shoulders to the whole family. We asked our other children to participate in being allergy advocates. Asking what was in things became the norm again, much like when Alex was a toddler and labels weren't reliable. We tipped waiters well who understood the whole allergy experience and honored and respected it and went over and beyond with their service. We asked for new waiters when we didn't feel heard or taken seriously.

I realized how far behind we were in preparing Alex to live with this, since I had so hopefully banked on him outgrowing it. Since the nature of homeschooling had kept him closer to us than he might have been had he left every day to head to school, I had not empowered him to handle it as much as I wanted him to immediately be able to. I had kept protection and control in my hands instead of training his self-preservation from age five onward. It was big work on his part to own the responsibility for his safety. Getting a nine-year-old boy to shower or to brush his teeth can be challenging; getting Alex to hold these peanut avoidance and safety related tasks was daunting.

Passing the Baton

Not only did he have to deal with the typical life skills, but he had his own special set of life skills dealing with his food allergy. There's a myriad of tasks that I nudged Alex into as I became intent on helping him navigate the landscape for himself. He needed to be able to jump over instead of stand terrified at the edge of each peanut related puddle that popped up in his path. It's hard to fully order your own food for the first time as a kid let alone if you are trying to educate the server or manager on your life-threatening food allergy.

Add to that any fear, shame, or anxiety you have about your allergy and imagine being able to make it seem serious to a stranger while feeling timid. Would you be able to truly gauge if that stranger got it or not while you were frozen inside with stage fright type feelings? It didn't feel great muttering your whole business to a stranger.

In these early days of trying to pass the baton to Alex, when he was asked about food by a stranger, he often froze at the task. I continued to model for him what to say. Kurt coached him through the trepidation. We gave voice to his difficulty every time it came up, and this meant anytime we left the house and encountered food. Basically, we got to practice this important food allergy life skill at least five times a week.

My younger kids, however, got into it. They were often braver to ask and converse with others than Alex was. It wasn't as heavy of a burden on them. I think he started to gain more confidence as he heard others say it, openly respect it, and talk about his food allergy besides me and one other person. The more he saw it was not dismissed, the more he gained confidence in bringing it up when needed. In all the years before when he had heard me asking questions related to his allergy, I am not sure he owned it. Perhaps he merely felt like a victim of some unknown evil I had shielded him from. I wanted him to hold the shield with me.

I think that Alex started from a young age in a tender place regarding his allergy. This is probably partly due to his personality and temperament and partly rooted in his life experiences. As a child, being singled out for something isn't ever preferred. Children who have a visible disability or difference want to be accepted and accommodated, but not singled out at every group gathering. They want tolerance and inclusion but not undue attention to their difference. While Alex's allergic condition isn't visible, he feels the same way. I imagine anyone with a hidden medical condition can understand this dynamic.

With food, this nuance of attention and accommodation versus normalcy and inclusion is tricky. Food holds such a sacred place in every culture. It is a way we commune; it is involved in most every activity humans do. There is also such a continuum of what people understand allergies to be. One person might say that they are allergic to onions but what they mean is they are digestively bothered by onions. So, when they hear that Alex is allergic to peanuts, they put their food discomfort, their food intolerance experience and understanding on top of what they hear about his allergy.

Others don't always equate allergy to anaphylaxis. They don't equate his allergy with a bullet wound that might not heal. They don't respect it the same, or respect it as they would someone that needed insulin or an inhaler to breathe or assistance walking. This leads to distrust and fear of people that might not mean any ill will at all. There isn't a universal language for allergy or reactions because it's different for everyone and anaphylaxis isn't always the result for everyone or understood.

When Alex shied away from conversation about his allergy, I think it was the memory of the prior reactions, a true fear in talking about an unpleasant event. I think he also desired to not be stared at by others, to not feel different, left out or excluded, to not feel that he was broken. In error, I catered to that. I kept the details and the seriousness between us adults, and I passed it on to other kids in private in simple terms. I largely talked about it out of Alex's earshot, even with my own younger kids. I was protective of Alex's emotions surrounding his allergy to a fault. Some of my handling of it in this way also stemmed from my thoughts that one day he would outgrow it and this would all be behind us. My handling of this morphed as my awareness and acceptance traveled further from his early childhood.

One event comes to mind that epitomizes the catch 22 of this allergy awareness dynamic. It was the summer after we had moved back to my hometown. We were in a safe feeling place. I knew lots of people from growing up in the neighborhood. Summer was in full swing when we arrived, and feeling nostalgic, I saw Alex enjoying the swim team like I had with my sisters growing up. Knowing the swim team coach, I took Alex to the first team meeting and practice of the season.

This gathering was full of children and adults communing on a festive summer day with candy and snacks others brought to share. One of the coaches, meaning only goodwill, stood up at the beginning and introduced Alex, telling everyone Alex was new to town, and that he was going to join the team. The coach, in hopes of keeping Alex safe and in making him feel safe with the team, loudly exclaimed to the group of over 75 kids, "Now I need you all to know, Alex is highly allergic to peanuts; if he eats something or touches something with peanuts on it, he could DIE. So, don't eat peanuts around him, everyone, let's make him feel safe!" Feeling called out like this sent Alex deep into his shell.

He survived the gathering, but I could sense his desire to flee. Needless to say, that was the end of swim team for Alex. He never wanted to go back to that exposed rock feeling he'd had on the first day. It was moments like these that peppered his childhood. I was grateful for the awareness in each moment and sad for the necessity. As we conversed about his feelings afterward, we were able to help him process them and feel more empowered in the future. Through these conversations, he gained traction in the ability to delicately balance shouting about his food allergy and guarding his privacy about it.

There were some rocky times in these years when I was asking Alex to be more mature regarding his allergy than might have seemed possible for a child. Family members found it difficult to control their panic as they watched and facilitated the passing of this responsibility to Alex. They had to learn to trust that Alex had asked sufficiently and learn their new role of mentoring him to ask and be safe rather than just keeping him safe themselves. We had asked them to keep him safe for so many years and now we were asking them to stand by calmly and watch him do it himself and only intervene if necessary.

I feel it was that unintentionally conveyed panicked fear from those of us that loved Alex the most and wanted desperately to keep him safe that made this transition so difficult. He didn't know if he could hold this scary responsibility that he had witnessed us all stressfully holding for years, let alone if he wanted to hold it while there were still loving adults that could do it instead. It was like learning to balance your checkbook when you didn't have the math skills of addition and subtraction under your belt yet.

When you trust someone else with your food, a stranger at a restaurant, you must be demanding or demonstrative but in a kind way to have your requests taken seriously. You must be able to trust a stranger to understand that your life is in their hands after an interaction that might be thirty seconds or just a few minutes. I got cards printed out that spelled out the reality and the seriousness of the allergy and the request to the server to handle his dish with caution. This way after a conversation, he could hand these to the server before he had all the words. It was a big deal to feel safe eating when it wasn't food from our house. Since Alex only had an allergy to one food, eating out was possible and was a part of his childhood. Practicing eating out safely was part of his past and present, and it was going to be a part of his future as an adult.

This passing of the baton also involved our family friends and Alex's friends. I got him to start asking the other parents or his friends the food questions. When others asked me what was or wasn't safe for Alex to eat, I involved Alex in that conversation before I answered. As much as I wanted to hold onto every shred of control and hope that I could prevent a reaction, I couldn't. When I considered Alex's whole adult future ahead of him with this allergy, it was a disservice if I mediated the difficulties and daily realities. To be able to live safely with it, he needed to have it every day in his face just like I had buffered it for eight years. It was here to stay, and he needed to navigate through the teen years and on into adulthood with his hands on the wheel.

CHAPTER 8 - FOURTH AND FIFTH BITES

This time our accident counter had gotten to about three years, over 1,000 days. Alex went from age eight to age eleven without a reaction. In the first week of December of 2010, we got a call saying that Alex's paternal great grandfather had entered a facility and was terminally ill. It was time for Kurt to go and say goodbye. Although the kids didn't know Kurt's grandfather well, we accompanied Kurt to South Dakota. As Kurt needed a second driver, me, to get there on time, we viewed it as an opportunity to have family time and see snow. We quickly packed up for a long road trip, and Kurt and I took turns driving over 20 hours there and back to say his goodbyes.

We were gone longer than a weekend and stayed in a hotel. It had a small waterpark in the lobby, but it was still a hotel. This meant lots of eating out and an inflammatory load on Alex's body. Being around the chlorine from the pool was stressful to his skin. The dry, cold winter air that wasn't our moist Alabama fall and winter was also a stressor.

Most of that time, I was alone with the kids while Kurt said goodbye to his grandfather and spent a few meals out with other adult family members. The kids and I holed up in the hotel and took breaks swimming, playing in the snow, or exploring the town of Sioux Falls. We were surprised to find a beautiful butterfly house in the middle of a snowstorm and a magical river walk downtown covered in icicles and snow. While we did have to eat out now and again, three quarters of our eating was from the mini fridge in the room that I stocked with food from the local grocery.

I headed to the grocery store again the third day we were there, when the food we had brought along had dwindled and the hotel meals had grown old, to get some easy to microwave supplies and fresh fruits. My newest and youngest daughter, just two years old, was in the grocery cart, and the older three kids were walking and shopping along with me as well as going off two by two to retrieve items from the shelves. It was like a scavenger hunt for them in this big, unfamiliar store.

This store had samples in the produce, deli, and bakery area. I recall stopping and sampling some pineapple, some grapes, and a piece of cheese. I was standing at the cooler case at the back of the store when Alex came to me wide eyed. "Mom," he said excitedly, "did you taste that spicy bread? It's really kind of good."

I froze, hearing those code red words again, and turned to face him. I had just walked the same store with him and sampled the same things, and there weren't any spicy breads that I knew of. Spicy was that old alarm bell for allergen that was stuck in my head from his two-year-old voice exclaiming spicy, spicy, spicy at Kurt's peanut butter sandwich. That moment jumped from deep within my brain to the forefront, flashing and honking and screeching the brakes on our shopping task.

I expressed my concern to Alex that a spicy taste in that bread could mean peanut and his face fell. I offered, "Let's go back and have you show me what bread you're talking about." We went back around the corner, and it was the banana bread that we had sampled. The banana bread did not have any peanuts in it, but it did contain walnuts. Alex had been eating walnuts as he got older. As he had gotten cleared by the allergist to eat all nuts except peanuts, we did eat nuts that didn't carry peanut warnings since by now food labeling was the law and much better than before. Since peanuts are a bean and not as closely related botanically to nuts as they are to soybeans and other legumes, he didn't have to restrict himself from other nuts, but when avoiding peanuts if there is cross contamination labeling, often other nuts are avoided, or they were in Alex's early life.

We talked there in the bakery area about how it had felt when he ate it and what his body was feeling right then. He told me his throat wasn't feeling great. We decided to go out to the quiet of the car where I could distract the other kids with the DVD player and assess if he was having a cross contamination reaction that was isolated to his throat or a full-blown beginning of an anaphylactic reaction. This was the first time I didn't know for sure that he'd ingested peanuts, but he was having similar symptoms.

I abandoned the cart there in the store and scurried with everyone back to the minivan. Back tucked warmly in the van, eye to eye with Alex in the front seat, it was apparent that this was a reaction. I went through the logic with him. If you know you have ingested something, and you are having one or two systems reacting you inject an *Epipen*. If you aren't sure you have ingested and you are having two systems reacting and escalating, you inject an *Epipen*.

He had escalating throat discomfort; likely, it was swelling. His chest felt tight, and I heard a noise that sounded like labored breathing. I talked about the logical next step that we needed to do, the *Epipen*, to be safe, and I asked him to do it if he could. He decided that he couldn't do it. He told me he would do it if I weren't there, but since he didn't have to, he didn't want to. We decided this time as a compromise to do it together. So, with my hand around his, there in a cold parking lot in South Dakota, Alex had his fourth administration of epinephrine.

As it had before, the reaction for him stopped pretty immediately, within minutes. This time his tears ceased quickly, and he looked up at me and said, "That wasn't as bad as I thought it was going to be. Each time it's easier. I think I'll be able to do it next time." Relief and grief washed over me. That was what I wanted to hear, that it would be easy one day for him to inject himself! And again that grief surfaced, recognizing that even as a child he knew, realized, and accepted that he would be doing it again one day, sooner rather than later. He was eleven years old and well on his to becoming a food allergy and *Epipen* expert.

At this point, I went against our food allergy action plan, making the executive decision not to drag everyone into the ER, either because of the cold or the fact that I was tired and miles from home alone with four children while Kurt said his goodbyes to his grandfather. This decision, while maybe not wise and definitely veering off our plan, was colored by thinking this reaction was cross contamination instead of a full peanut product dose.

My decision to not enter the ER was not a complete disregard for safety. I did decide to get some food for the kids at a drive thru, and we sat finishing the movie in the car in the parking lot of the nearby ER. If anything had escalated in the next hour, I would have been right there to rush Alex inside. Nothing else came of it, and we soon went back to the hotel for the night.

In South Dakota while Alex's great grandfather's life was ending, Alex earned one more skill set about saving his own life. I moved quicker this fourth time from the guilt to the grace to the gratitude that the spicy banana bread had happened on my watch. Nothing was an accident anymore if I could color it and memorialize it as a boost of knowledge for a future accidental ingestion.

A New Allergy Addition

After reacting to the banana bread, I took Alex in for testing when we were back at home. I wanted to make sure that there wasn't a new allergy to walnuts that had caused his reaction instead of peanut cross contamination. Our local allergist did not do bloodwork for walnut, but she did order skin testing. I think now that I should have challenged that clinical decision and requested a blood test as well, or a supervised food challenge, but I didn't.

Alex's skin tests came back highly positive for walnut. Under the allergist's advice, we added walnut allergy to his peanut allergy, and from that point forward, we followed all the same protocols for walnut that we did for peanut. We got to learn where walnuts hid in our food lives, not in as many places as peanut, but in some surprising ones. Food avoidance got a little stricter and food choices narrowed slightly adding walnut allergy to the list.

Curry Disaster

Thirteen months later in January 2012, we were headed home from a day celebrating our daughter, Emma's, dragon artwork that had been chosen for display at the Birmingham Museum of Art in their Chinese Year of the Dragon celebration. Having a food allergy restriction hadn't made Alex afraid of any other kind of food except peanuts and now walnuts. He was an adventurous eater, always willing to eat more food options than most adults I knew. I think because there were so many things that he couldn't eat, he was always up for eating anything that he knew was safe.

He will eat the spiciest pepper. He will make odd food combinations just to see what they taste like. His allergy could have given him reservations and pickiness about food, but it swung the other way. He has a voracious appetite for food novelty. He is usually willing to try anything, beef tongue, raw sushi, you name it. The normal constraints of tasting bad or having bad texture aren't what informs his choice not to eat something. Only the fear of reaction, only the known allergen danger made him say no to eating a food.

He loved odd, he loved new, he loved sushi, he loved spicy. If he trusted that we or he could ask for it to be prepared safely, he was up for trying it. As a child, we would have never eaten at some restaurants with Alex; everything when he was younger was more black and white and restrictive. But as that child we were protecting grew older and the scales of avoidance started to balance with the reality and freedom of him living a full life, constraints had loosened. Now, he could verbalize and know if something wasn't right if he ate it.

Food culture and food allergy education and safety had also come a long way since Alex was little. Restaurants had special menus or icons for gluten free and allergy eating. Many had policies in place to ask or notify your server if you had a food allergy. More chefs and managers had training in accommodating food allergy diners. So, Alex's horizons were wider, and we allowed him to take advantage of all that he could and would.

The three of us knew what a reaction entailed at this point. We knew Alex could handle it, and we also knew that it would happen again one day, even if we stayed safely locked in the house or never ate food prepared by anyone else. That wasn't the life we wanted for Alex, but we also didn't want him to navigate his first years of autonomous food choice alone as a teen and adult without a few good years of navigating that reality with us at his side. It was better to try the new ice cream place and watch them clean the blenders for his shake and use clean scoops and new ice cream containers while we were there with him than to know he would one day try that on his own as a young adult with a group of friends.

Many restaurants that we couldn't go to when Alex was a child were now places we went with Alex as an older child and teenager. Alex wanted to learn to eat out safely at any places he reasonably could. He didn't eat at places with peanut shells and crumbs or peanut oil on all the surfaces, but he had already experienced eating out at places that served peanuts somewhere on their menu already.

That January day on the way home, the kids chose to eat at a chain Asian fusion restaurant. They probably chose this because we were celebrating the Chinese New Year. This wasn't our first time dining at an Asian restaurant. We had eaten at other places and had experience with asking for Alex's dish to be cooked in a separate, clean wok or pan and in asking detailed questions about ingredients.

If you have a small child that has a peanut allergy, you might be saying in your head, you ate at an Asian restaurant; are you out of your mind; they have peanuts there! And if you're an adult with a peanut allergy, you might also declare you would never eat at that type of restaurant either. So, I understand that to some this choice might appear negligent. But for Alex, we wanted his food world to be as big as it could be because experience had proven to us that even keeping it small and safe and to only the familiar didn't guarantee safety. We read the tragic stories of an adult eating curry or some other dish and dying. We wanted to be around as Alex navigated the loosening of some of his dietary restrictions, as he felt confident trying peanut avoidance more places. We thought if he was like most anyone else, he would inevitably experiment with more food choices as an invincible young adult outside of our home. We knew that reactions weren't to be feared as much as they were to be avoided, prepared for, recognized and acted upon quickly.

We stopped at the chain restaurant off the interstate on the way home. Alex chose to get a spicy curry rice dish. Spicy foods were often his favorites. The waiter was informed of the peanut allergy, the severity, and asked if he understood the difference between an allergy like this versus a food preference like requesting no tomatoes on a salad. He assured us he understood and would alert the manager. The curry sauce was also checked by the server and manager for any peanut ingredients, and they ensured that Alex's dish was made in a clean skillet or pan. Everything went as smoothly as it had in similar spots and situations.

Our family chatted waiting for our food. There were the usual distractions you'd expect while dining with four children under the age of 12: walking around the restaurant, coloring pages, getting an item from the car, stopping at the bathroom, and playing on an electronic device. It was the middle of the afternoon and not busy at all, so it wasn't long before the food came. We all started devouring.

I did a check in with Alex after he started eating. He exclaimed it was delicious. We ate on. Alex is a fast eater; he reminds me of my dad, they can both engulf some food. I'm such a slow eater. I'm always stunned at how fast they finish. A couple of minutes later, probably halfway through his curry, Alex spoke up with a tone of regret in his voice. "Mom, I think that the spicy taste I was enjoying is maybe more than just the curry being spicy because I don't feel really well; my stomach hurts all of a sudden and my throat feels icky. This might have peanut in it."

The meal ended for Alex and me immediately. We went out to the parking lot into the sun and fresh air to assess. His eyes had that panicked look that toddler Alex had before. This is the look of doom that allergy warning posters talk about. I think, for Alex, it's a mood change and a more dilated look to his pupils, which isn't a result of worry but rather a physical change happening in his body. I asked him to take a deep breath and go through the body systems to see how he was feeling.

That brave, food allergy expert twelve-year-old did it. He calmed down as he ticked off the symptoms. My stomach hurts, like I could throw up; that's not normal. My throat feels irritated; that's not normal for spicy food when I eat it. This is a place they do serve peanuts; my allergen is there in the kitchen so despite what training they had and what we requested, there could have been a mistake made. I asked him if he knew what was next. He said, "Yes, I don't want to do it, but I know it can't hurt me to use the *Epipen*, so I should do it now before it's too late. But, I'm afraid to because I think it'll make me vomit how I'm feeling right now, but I know I must do it." His eyes were teary, but he was aware and committed.

Then that brave kid asked me to count with him, and he gave himself his *Epipen* right there in the parking lot. Sure, enough he did get sick. Who knows why he vomited this time instead of other times. The amount of allergen? The type of food? He did have an adult size *Epipen* by this time because of his weight, so the new amount of epinephrine and what that did in his body could have affected him differently. We had been told by our allergist that vomiting was not a bad thing; if it did happen, it would get the allergen out of his system quickly.

So, he had succeeded: his first self-injection of epinephrine. I got on the phone with the allergist after this to ask her advice based on the fact we were out of town. I wanted to know if we should call an ambulance, proceed to an ER, or go to the ER in our town that was just about as far away. She talked to Alex on the phone, and we decided which ER to head towards and what to look for to administer another *Epipen* in route if needed.

Surprisingly, this event, again, did not send Alex into more fear and more avoidance. There was a period where he didn't eat curry and only chose sushi at restaurants like this. But, he eventually went back to choosing to eat anything he could and advocating for his safety when warranted. It made him more confident and assured of what to do in the event of a reaction as he had experienced self-administering his *Epipen* for the first time. I learned later this same year there had been a recall issued for curry seasoning that had similar looking peanut flour added as a filler, which wasn't disclosed on the ingredients. We added curry seasoning as a possible contamination to avoid unless the spice integrity could be verified. I suspected this could have been the mystery as to what happened that day as the manager could find no peanut contamination in any of the steps they took to make Alex's curry dish.

I sat there on the ride home that night holding regret, guilt, and doubt once again. What kind of idiot was I that we ever let him eat anywhere but at home? And then I circled back around to the reality of his world and future that wouldn't always be in my home, partly because I had no choice in protecting him forever, and needed to give everything a positive spin to continue to put one foot in front of the other in as healthy a way as possible, and partly because I believed it to be true. I chose again to find the good in this incident. I focused on hope that he was getting all the steady walking legs he'd need to live life alone one day with his allergy.

CHAPTER 9 - SEARCHING AND RESEARCHING

Planning for the Future

I had known since Alex was eight that he wasn't outgrowing this allergy. The idea of your eight-year-old not living at home one day is a reality for most everyone, but at the time it was esoteric. This eight-year-old of mine was my oldest child, and I had three younger kids now as well. Anyone of them leaving home and living on their own seemed so far away and part of fantasy futuristic world, I couldn't picture it. Regarding preparing Alex for his food allergy in his life away from home, I pieced together ideas from everywhere into a big melting pot, hoping I was covering all the bases.

As Alex got older, grew taller than me, and went away to summer camps for several weeks, I tried to see his future more clearly. Some parents might focus on career, gap years, jobs, internships, college and all the other things young adults do as they leave home. I held those thoughts, too, just not as intensely as I thought about him living alone with his food allergies.

I saw articles about teens and their food allergy challenges that hadn't been on my radar before, kind of like you see pregnant people everywhere once you are pregnant or wanting to be. New questions and worries surfaced that hadn't concerned me before. What if Alex kissed someone that had eaten peanuts earlier that day? Not only did teens with food allergies have the normal jitters at a first kiss with someone, but they would also have jitters over needing to ask if it was safe food-wise to kiss?

It seemed like every few months there was an article about some teen or adult who had a fatal anaphylactic reaction. I read speculation on whether teens increased risk was due to changes in hormones and how their body reacted; the reality of teens being apt to take more risks and brush off the severity of a reaction; increased independence making more opportunities for accidental ingestion; or more time without supervision by a parent, a friend, or a teacher that knew of their allergy.

I pored over these stories of teens and young adults who lost their lives to a food allergy reaction, trying to pick out what had gone wrong on that one ingestion after they had survived their whole childhood. It was a sick, dark thing to do, but I obsessed a bit over each story. I thought I could learn from these tragedies and honor those who had lost their lives to a food allergy in a small way by preventing another loss of life from a food allergy reaction. I searched for something to pass on to Alex that he didn't already know that might save his life if his next reaction were different. If as a teen or an adult, he was alone.

I remember telling Alex that I needed to have a serious conversation with him. When we sat down to talk, I didn't sugarcoat anything; I laid all my fears out. He was almost 15, and he has always been a mature soul, so I knew he could hear and talk to me like an adult. He could hear the dire and the real fear in our chat and not crumble. I told him that I loved him and my goal was to keep him safe. As he was getting older and older, it seemed harder and harder for me to figure out. I told him about the news stories of teens, young adults, and grown adults who had lost their lives because of an allergen reaction that had gone untreated too long or failed for an unknown reason.

I shared with him that I wanted him to feel terrified enough to take it seriously and know that he wasn't invincible, but also live without fear. I admitted I worried I was screwing that possibility up by scaring him, but I also thought some fear might act as a coping and safety mechanism. At the end of the conversation, we sat and read some of the news stories together from news reports, blogs, and websites that memorialized victims of food allergy anaphylaxis. I wished him to hear and know all that I did. I read these stories out loud, with tear filled eyes. He listened and hugged me tightly occasionally.

We brainstormed that day how to get through these years of passing responsibility from us to him. I told him this was a burden no child should have to carry, but he did have it, and he did need to carry it. I told him he was strong, he was built for struggle and beautiful things could come of struggle, and I believed in him succeeding. I think that after this long emotional chat, a switch flipped inside of Alex. After that, he took a more active, decisive role. All our struggles with him carrying his *Epipen* and remembering to carry his *Epipen* fell away. He became less forgetful of those tasks that had always been a struggle. He was on board and responsible in a way that hadn't happened before.

He initiated conversations with servers and folks that offered and brought food to potlucks. All the shyness about advocating and announcing his food allergy was gone. I was in awe. I was proud of him. But, I was heartbroken that I had laid out in such detail the reality that he could die, and that I needed him to know that and hold it as much as I did so that he could keep himself safe. Could I have had this or a similar conversation earlier? I don't know. When he was a child, I didn't ever consider telling him through black and white analogies and other people's stories that this was life or death. It was known but had never been spoken about as starkly. Abstractly, Alex as a child knew that he could stop breathing and that his life depended on it, but he'd never heard a real-life recounting of another teen, child or adult, to the best of my knowledge, losing their life to an accidental ingestion.

Alex's local allergist also helped his understanding at his annual checkup to get his epinephrine prescription refilled. I asked her to please talk about the realities and procedures again regarding anaphylaxis with Alex like it was the first day he was learning of his allergy and like he was an adult. She agreed to my request and did a professional job at that visit, talking to him and educating him more than she had on any of his other allergy visits growing up.

Researching OIT

I was hopeful one day there would be something to try for Alex's allergy. There had been murmurings for years of peanut allergy prescriptions or cures on the horizon. I believe I first heard of Oral Immunotherapy for food allergies in 2014. I know that it was towards the end of the year and after Alex and I had our long allergy chat. I read an article that I found on someone's Facebook feed about trials happening regarding immunotherapy and desensitizing people to peanuts.

Luckily, peanuts are and have always been a highly studied allergen. If there's a trial or a research study about food allergies, it likely has peanuts as one of the foods being studied. I was often sent links and articles about things relating to peanut allergy whether it was about something as obscure as parasites curing people to news of the peanut patch on the horizon. I read everything I came across. I checked it with Alex's allergist at yearly appointments, but nothing seemed concrete.

This article I saw in 2014 about Oral Immunotherapy was different. There were trials that you could get into with links listed. This was my first introduction to OIT: hearing randomly of it as something that happened in trials. Later, I hoped for a trial near us in Atlanta or in Vanderbilt maybe. In this process of searching, I didn't find trials nearby that Alex qualified for but I came across a

Michigan allergist's website who practiced OIT and got excited for the possibility of traveling to do OIT there. The website I stumbled upon was OITCenter[7], the site of the office of Dr. Chad W. Mayer, an allergist in Michigan. I called Dr. Mayer's office to confirm this treatment was available, and the receptionist gave me helpful information, inviting me to a consultation.

Kurt and I talked it over, and knowing that with Alex's age he would need to consent for any treatment, I went to Alex to explain what I knew of OIT, the doctor I had found and asked if he would be willing to travel and explore it. I was surprised at his reaction. He was adamant that in no way was he interested in eating his allergen under doctor's supervision to become desensitized. He wasn't even interested in going to an appointment or a consultation to learn more about it with no commitment required.

At this point, I backed off. It had to be his choice; he wasn't 5, so I couldn't sneak oral immunotherapy or other protocols on him. I abandoned my first exploration and knowledge of OIT quickly. I did ask Alex to keep the idea of OIT in his head as he went about life, and when an issue related to his allergy came up, he should think how it could be different if he weren't allergic at the same level or amount anymore. I told him I couldn't understand how scared he might feel to eat his allergen intentionally, but I did ask him to think about what it could mean to be desensitized.

Not everyone with a lifetime diagnosis of something gets an opportunity to reverse, or at least reverse the effects of fear and anxiety, a condition they are born with. I expressed that he should consider it for that reason alone because he could. I shared that as his mom, the idea that he could possibly live in the world safer without the fear of dying from an accidental ingestion seemed like a miracle. I was honest and told him it was hard to hear him give such a quick no to exploring what OIT would be like, but that I respected it and wouldn't bring it up again, at least not for a while. Thus, OIT went on the back burner at our house to simmer and percolate for consideration another year.

I wish I could go back to the moment I found that article on Facebook about OIT and find the person who shared it, the journalist who wrote it, the editor who approved it, the family who agreed to be interviewed, and the allergist who provided the process and take them all out for a night on the town. That share was a needle in a haystack that I didn't even know I was searching for.

During 2015, I binged and immersed myself in long Internet searches about Oral Immunotherapy for food allergies. I read research articles from the trial studies, and every article and blogpost I could find on the research statistics on these same trial studies. I read countless blogs of parents that were in OIT with their kids. Towards the end of the year, I found every Facebook group regarding OIT and lurked and read posts back from months and months prior.

Two Facebook groups, both OIT101 and Private Practice OIT, were instrumental in giving me a community and access to resources to help make the leap to OIT. I had been out of food allergy parent groups for so long since I no longer craved additional knowledge and support once Alex was older. Because food allergy lives were different since I had hunted for hope in the early 2000s, there was a lot to digest.

On these pages, I found specifics on the process of doing OIT outside of a trial setting and outside of an in-theory conversation in a news article. I read how it worked undergoing OIT with a trained Private Practice OIT (PP OIT) Allergist. Much of what I found on these pages has now migrated and grown into the website I recommended in the forward of this book, www.oit101.org. In these groups, I found files and documents to pour over. I found a directory of PP OIT allergists, some that were near me, closer than Michigan. I didn't hesitate to google the three nearby doctors and pour over their credentials and histories.

I want to clarify the science of OIT so there is not any misunderstanding on OIT being a cure for food allergy. It is a food allergy treatment that does cure the social and emotional impact of food allergy avoidance, but it does not cure food allergy in the body. After one finishes OIT, you are technically still allergic to your allergen; you will just be desensitized up to a certain amount. The OIT website explains it best:

"The key to understanding OIT is that there is low level of allergen an allergic person can safely eat without a reaction. It's invisible to the body. Then it's raised slightly and the body still doesn't react. The "threshold of tolerance" is gradually increased over time. The immune and digestive systems adapt, as they are meant to do.

The treatment process can take 6-12 months with 15-25 "updoses" reaching a daily serving of the allergen being eaten with no symptoms. After a period, usually 3 months to 12 months at this dose, there is a final "challenge" of about double or triple what the daily amount is (i.e. a 20-peanut challenge when eating 10/day). This challenge simulates "unlimited" eating and that the patient is "fully desensitized" to their allergen. From that point, you go into maintenance where X amount per day is eaten to keep the body recognizing the allergen.

For many, the dosing will continue for life. Perhaps not daily, but regularly like 3-5 times a week in a normal diet." (OIT101, 2016b).

About a year after I had first asked Alex about considering OIT, I asked him again. This time he said sure, it couldn't hurt to check it out. He had changed his mind. I didn't waste a moment. I think that by the end of this same day that Alex said yes, I had made consultation appointments with all three of the private practice OIT allergists near us. I also found their patient only Facebook pages, if they had one, where I could see and ask the nitty gritty of current patients at each practice.

OIT is not new, but it is a unique, real-time active medical conversation. I was elated to see that online there were parents and allergists and other professionals discussing the ins and outs of OIT, the fears and what ifs. The particulars of their experience were shared with complete strangers. It was like being transported back to a breastfeeding support group that I had been a part of as a new mom. There was a melding of keeping the medical and particulars of the protocol specific to each patient and only within the trained allergists' hands. But this existed along with a completely free space to discuss everything important with other people that understood what it was like.

I became aware in all my OIT research of a divide in the food allergy community over the use and promotion of OIT. Having not been on any allergy groups since the advent of social media, I didn't understand all the secrecy in some allergy circles and allergists who took the position to not mention OIT or share information about OIT. Having lived fifteen years with no options, I was grateful to be told of an option to explore. If someone had not shared OIT online, I wouldn't have had the option of exploring it.

Through my early lurking on the OIT groups, I learned that "OIT is not for everyone." I think that is the succinct phrase that a moderator on the page used. Whether that statement refers to the 5 to 15% that Private Practice OIT cannot help or whether it refers to the patients who can't complete the process for financial, travel, fear, or commitment to the protocol reasons. It is the truth: it's not for everyone; there's not anything that's best or feasible for everyone. On the oit101 website, Dr. Factor of the New England Food Allergy Treatment Center is quoted as saying, "The choice by patients and parents is a personal one, and a lot of thought must go into deciding whether OIT is right for them/their child" (OIT101, 2016c).

I do hold hope that OIT will one day be within anyone's reach if they want to try it. The more private practice allergists who get trained to offer OIT, the more allergic individuals will try it. There are already over 70 board certified allergists offering OIT in private practice in the United States. If you can overcome the travel and the financial burdens that exist with the OIT protocol and where it's offered now, then it's the only fear left to hurdle. Those with food allergies and parents of kids with food allergies are already living with fear.

I knew Alex would likely have another accidental ingestion, life had shown me that. So anything that made that future ingestion safer I was up for. My ultimate decision was based on the fact that OIT has a proven 85% success rate and up, and an even higher than 90% success rate in some doctor's personal records, so the odds were in Alex's favor.

I didn't escape all waffling back and forth though. If it was so safe and so effective, why wasn't everyone doing it? Repeatedly, I seemed to encounter the same set of refrains: Offering an individual protocol isn't possible in many allergist offices; it requires a different sort of commitment and availability on the part of the allergist; it couldn't be approved by the FDA; it was just eating your allergen in an individualized protocol; it was a series of food challenges over time; Private Practice OIT didn't make anyone any big money; it didn't lead to a prescription of the peanut patch or a pill; it takes a lot of time and effort to travel and do OIT; some teens and adults that have lived life so far learning to deal with their allergy can't see the benefit of trying at this point. None of the reasons I found to not try it held up to the intuition, the research, and the consultations that we eventually had.

This was not the first time I'd encountered something as a parent that was against the grain, that wasn't in the majority. I wasn't afraid to do an out of the box move. When I asked our local allergist about OIT, she didn't know all that I knew. She said what many allergists say: it was something happening in research trials for a peanut patch, that it wasn't safe, that it wasn't a real hope for Alex. I just listened and knew I would stack what she said against the three allergists, who were just as qualified as she, whom I was about to consult with.

At some point my analytical side plateaued. I couldn't take any more data in, or taking in more data didn't sway me either way. In order to intuit which path to take, I had to physically talk to the private practice OIT allergists, see their results, and hear their experiences.

I didn't choose an OIT allergist as much as I chose to go to the ones closest to us. The closest city with a private practice OIT allergist had three of them. So, to eliminate all doubt, I chose to take Alex to visit and consult with all three. I figured the $200 consultation fee, if insurance didn't cover it for all three, was worth it to know for sure whom we wanted to go with. I secured all three consultations on two days back to back about three weeks away. I had lived without any hope regarding food allergy for 15 years, and in a matter of a month, I had hope and an appointment to meet and shake hope's hand!

CHAPTER 10 - CONSULTATIONS

As the consultation dates approached, we had many tasks to complete. I dredged up Alex's old records from out of state and prior allergists. I got new labs ordered that the OIT doctors requested. I sent off emails, faxes, and mailings to all three offices with labs and history. We were full of hope and excitement at the appointments coming up.

Alex had to go and get new labs drawn to see where his "numbers" were. Since the last time he had labs ordered, there was a new test related to peanut allergy, the ImmunoCAP Peanut Component Allergen Test. This test according to Quest Laboratories description "helps to assess a patient's level of risk of a life-threatening reaction, and may reassure patients when the risk for allergic symptoms is low or when they will most likely experience mild or localized reactions upon exposure to peanut. The test helps the health care provider identify primary, species-specific allergic sensitization, differentiate between symptoms caused by a primary allergen source and those caused by cross-reactivity, assess the level of risk for life-threatening allergic reactions, and provide clarity regarding the patient's risk of an allergic reaction to ease fears and help target effective management" (2000).

This test looks at reactivity to five peanut proteins: Ara h 2, Ara h 1, Ara h 3, Ara h 9, and Ara h 8. Results can inform the allergist of the type of reaction a patient might have if they have never had a reaction or the type of reaction a patient that hasn't reacted in a while might have. It provides more data for better allergy management decisions.

This was a new test that I didn't even know existed! I wondered, in the back of my mind, why Alex's allergist, whom he sees yearly, had not recommended this test earlier to give us more information on his allergy. Perhaps it was a matter of it not being a standard lab covered by insurance at the time. The private practice OIT allergists requesting more labs than what our local allergist had ordered in the past boosted my confidence that we were doing the right thing by searching out answers to food allergy from doctors working with cutting edge processes and protocols.

Alex hadn't had his blood drawn in five years, so he got to experience that process as more of an adult. He told the lab tech when he was ready for the needle to go in. This was the first thing regarding OIT that gave Alex back a bit of his humanity and dignity, healing the consent boundaries that had been broken when he was so tiny.

He had been given *Epipens* 3 times without his full consent. The violence inherent in having to quickly inject him with epinephrine was finally in reparation. It was healing for me as a mom, who had no choice in those accidental ingestions but to hold him tight and inject him against his will, to finally get to apologize for that not just in words but in actionable moments. With everything regarding OIT, he was calling the shots.

Consultation day was upon us. I had scheduled the consults over two days on our spring break. We had one appointment on Monday afternoon and two on Tuesday, one morning and one afternoon. We planned to stay overnight in a hotel between the two offices, and then head to our vacation on the coast for the rest of the week. Our two teens were also touring a college on our vacation.

I didn't go into these appointments blind. I'd been online for weeks nonstop, cramping my hand and neck typing and reading on tiny mobile screens. For two of the three doctors we were visiting, I had already questioned their current patients via the online groups and seen what others had experienced. I read articles about each doctor. I was over prepared.

We created a list of questions for the allergists. Alex added his questions to the list. One of his questions stood out to me: "How do you get over the fear of eating your allergen." I was interested to see how the allergist answered that very non-clinical question. I knew that as we sat in each office and looked into the allergist's eyes, we would know what to ask, and could decide if we felt like considering doing OIT with that office.

It pretty much went like I expected. I think after all my research and lurking and reading on the other parent's experiences, I already knew which direction I wanted to go. However, I wanted it to be

Alex's choice and have Kurt's input, and I was open to being wrong on my preference. Sometimes things look glossier online than they are in person. Sometimes I can read and intuit things through printed word, and other times, I need to see it with my own two eyes to gauge. All vetted private practice OIT allergists are valid places to do OIT. I knew that, but I wanted to choose after an in-person visit.

The first allergist spent time going over Alex's labs and gave us handouts about how the OIT process works. He then gave us his recommendation for Alex. He told us that based on history and labs that he would first recommend a food challenge of walnut since current labs on that allergen were at zero, despite the past incident in South Dakota and the prior positive skin test. He also advised starting OIT for peanut desensitization. He explained each protocols timeline and what would happen during both events. He left us to talk and formulate any questions telling us that we were welcome to stay as long as we wanted, no rush. He left to go and see a few patients and came back in to talk later.

I took a deep breath after he left the room. I had met a board certified OIT doctor. They had seemed almost mythical online. This was a regular board-certified allergist just like our allergist at home. Only he didn't look at me like I was from Mars and dismiss the idea of treating Alex's peanut allergy through oral immunotherapy.

I was a bit shocked. Seeing Oral Immunotherapy for food allergy made it real. This wasn't online isolated quackery. This wasn't alternative or unsafe medical care. This was a different form of the allergy injections I'd had as a child for pollen, grass, and environmental allergens. It was just now happening for food orally, too, and more widespread than just in trials.

We each assessed what the other thought and asked our own questions. I wanted to know why there seemed to be so many young kids at his practice and not teens; Alex asked his question about getting over the fear of eating his allergen for the food challenge and the first OIT visit; and Kurt questioned why do a food challenge at all, it seemed insane. I felt we were in his house on his sofa, and he kept coming back into the room for more questions between his other patients.

I'm not sure we stayed as long as we meant to. The visit felt shorter than a consultation for something of such magnitude. This wasn't due to lack of information or diligence on the allergist's part, but rather because in reality it was a simple protocol to explain at the outset. It was such a shock. A food challenge? Start OIT as soon as today or tomorrow? The allergist had no doubts at all it would work based on Alex's history, labs, and age. Really? We left the appointment to go get the other kids and spent our night processing, staying open to the same or new information at our next consultation.

Consultation number two was bright and early the next morning. The receptionist greeted us by name when we came in and asked how our trip had gone. Right from the beginning, I felt expertly cared for. This second allergist was calm and steadily talked about OIT with detailed knowledge and rationalization. He had a zen presence that put me at ease. He stayed with us the whole appointment, going over all of Alex's labs and pulled up research and labs from OIT studies to compare things as he explained. He wanted to hear a detailed history of each of Alex's reactions. He talked directly to Alex as the patient, not just to us, his parents. He asked Alex what exactly he was anxious about with OIT, and then had a conversation with him that addressed that fear.

We talked about food allergies in general, their prevalence, theories he had for that, what the future of allergy likely held. I liked this allergist's take on food allergy science. I got the sense that he was about fixing the problems of allergy with a viewpoint from the causation end of things as well as the treatment end. This allergist's advice didn't differ greatly from the first consultation: he also was certain OIT would work for Alex and recommended a food challenge for both nuts prior to OIT to make certain that the time and effort and lifelong maintenance dose of peanut or walnut were warranted. He explained this recommendation was based on the change in Alex's labs over his life and other factors in his reaction history. He explained how food challenges were the gold standard and lots of allergists didn't do them because they weren't trained in that setting, monitoring and facilitating them. He went through what a food challenge would be like. While he agreed to doing OIT for peanut without a food challenge, he recommended trying it as a food challenge first. The food challenge could then be converted into the beginning of peanut OIT if it didn't work.

This new idea of Alex food challenging peanut as well as walnut was a shock to us. If the food challenge idea at the first consult wasn't shocking enough, now this allergist recommended food challenging both things that our allergist had told us to avoid. It was perplexing. He gave us some time to talk. I would guess that we had been there about an hour already. He left to go and start an OIT appointment with another patient in the office and came back shortly. We all looked around at each other, and it seemed like a unanimous yes between us. This office and allergist felt like the place and the person to start OIT. Yes, we liked him; yes he got it; yes I could trust and see myself putting Alex's life and path on this food allergy treatment in his hands. Sometimes you just know what to do, this was one of those times.

When this allergist came back, he asked Alex if he could show him something. He wanted Alex to visually see something. He asked if he could do a quick skin test on Alex's arm to give him a visual marker of what was possible based on his lab results and change in skin reactions over time. Alex agreed. We then had a 30-minute wait to see how the welts for walnut and peanut and the control spot for histamine reacted. It was stunning. The peanut and walnut didn't react at all on the skin test.

This added even more complexity to the OIT decision. Our allergist every year had told Alex to continue avoiding these nuts, without retesting skin and rerunning labs after a certain age. As we conversed with this new allergist, our local allergist was going down notches in my book. This new allergist said it was possible Alex could have outgrown his peanut allergy since his last reaction, and we wouldn't know it if we didn't try. His labs were low, and labs could be medically right. The peanut component test did indicate positive reaction to the proteins with a more severe reaction correlation, but the numbers were on the low end. He explained that both high and low numbers were valid for severe allergy, but it would be valuable to know for sure. The food challenge was explained again as the gold standard since the lab numbers were low and a span of time had passed since Alex's last reaction.

At this point, the allergist explained some of the science of labs and their fallibilities, most of which was over my head. This was clearly not a doctor looking to make a year's worth of visits of money from us. He was advocating for us to make sure OIT was even necessary for both of Alex's food allergens before going further. That curry reaction could have been the last reaction; there was still some hope Alex had outgrown his allergy in the past four years. I was stunned.

Then we addressed Alex's question and had a big conversation about how to get into the right mental state to do a food challenge. He explained why he didn't do blind food challenges with people of Alex's age. The mindset he advised for Alex was to look at the labs, to look at the research, to look at the skin test as being negative; and to listen to the doctor's experience and wisdom and truth that he wouldn't recommend if he didn't have some measure of confidence he would pass. He wanted Alex to convince himself that he might not be allergic in order to enter a food challenge with hope instead of anxiety overriding everything. We soaked this all in. We thanked the allergist and headed out for a late breakfast and brunch with the rest of the family.

At this point, I was wiped out mentally. We had come for three consults for OIT, and at two consults in, we were being asked to consider food challenges and the possibility that Alex wasn't allergic at all anymore, that he'd possibly outgrown in the past four years! It was more than I could process anymore that day. Against everything that is in my nature, as I am not one to cancel plans without a reason, I decided there at brunch to cancel our third consult later that afternoon. There were several reasons, all valid.

I called the third allergist's office. I was honest with the assistant that answered. I told her that we had reached our limit with two consults already. Driving across town in traffic for another office visit was daunting. I said we would still pay for the consultation fee due to my cancelling last minute. But, they didn't want us to pay. So, we let that third consult go. I felt the two consults we had under our belt were enough to decide to proceed or not.

I am grateful the third allergist's staff heard my honesty and chose to not charge us and said it was no big deal at all to have the space open on the day's calendar. This alleviated my guilt. I think we made the right intuitive decision to not tackle another consult. That third one just wasn't meant to happen as a part of our exploration of OIT.

We left town driving towards our vacation for a week of bike rides, walks in the campground, romps on the beach, exploration of the city, a college tour, a city history tour, more good food than I can count and digesting all the future OIT held. Alex and Kurt and I had some conversations that were tinged with hope. We decided to not decide until we were back home.

Each OIT conversation felt like hopeful, upbeat uncertainty. This was foreign territory. Before these consults, any allergy conversations were based on facts and decisions were based on the most certain way to control the outcome and protect my child. I hadn't hoped for a life without his food allergy in a long time nor had I ever lived knowing he wasn't allergic or made effectively "bite-safe" to his allergen.

If he passed the food challenges, then that was it: our son wasn't allergic anymore despite what the labs said and what had happened in the past. If he passed both food challenges, all the stress of living with a food allergy would be gone in one moment. If he was still anaphylactic, then there was a clear path that both these OIT experienced allergists felt certain was going to work. It was like being handed a gift. We just had to decide to accept the gift and when and if we were ready to open it up.

CHAPTER 11 - A FOOD CHALLENGE

After our vacation, we sat down to decide. Before the consults, the decision to do OIT or not seemed difficult, but after being with each allergist, it was an easier decision. I'd read everything there was to read. We'd seen, grilled, and been advised by two top doctors with great OIT success. I already knew what life was like not doing OIT, we'd been doing that for 16 years. I knew Alex would likely have another ingestion and reaction at some point.

For me, it boiled down to deciding to take this path with more certainty. The outcome of OIT seemed more known; it felt like an active decision, like responding. Choosing not to do OIT and instead avoid the allergen had more unknowns, it felt like a passive decision, reacting out of fear. I wanted to have the most knowledge and certainty that I could give Alex in his life going forward. I wanted to release the illusion that I could control this, and instead, let these allergy experts manage a food allergy outcome with greater freedom and less fear and anxiety.

My decision to start OIT for Alex was a classic decision of love versus fear. A mentor of mine, Paul Nobrega, whom I met at a seminar in 2010, gave me the perspective of parsing a decision into its simplest terms to always choose love: "The two primary forces in the world are fear and love. One of the two is always behind whatever we do. At times, it's very subtle; other times, it's obvious. Yet it is nearly always one of the two pushing me along. Fear usually shows up in the following behaviors - reacting vs. responding, putting up walls instead of boundaries, being stuck in the victim role, and manipulation. Love usually shows up in the following behaviors - responding instead of reacting, putting up boundaries instead of walls, finding one's accountability, and releasing control. These forces are in a constant battle for dominance in our lives, and virtually every day we're are faced with choice points on which way we will go. Of course, the challenge is that we are usually not aware of the choice due to our own blind spots. Yet they are there. If we want love to win out more often than fear, it's important to train ourselves to identify those choice points when they come up, and then re-train ourselves to respond in love, and not react in fear. Of course, this can be very challenging - yet it's very doable."

With this mind frame, I knew walking away from OIT felt like a choice made from fear. Trying OIT felt like handing him love. That was the heart of it after stripping all the analysis and detail away. I wanted to try something that felt different than fear.

Alex was a go. Kurt was a go. I was a go. I am acutely aware that of the three of us, I felt the most anxiety about my yes. Mainly because I was the one that had brought this idea to the table, and I doubted I would ever forgive myself if it didn't work. One day at a time is how I breathed myself through the anxiety. I made the call to tell our chosen allergist, Dr. Agrawal, that we had decided to proceed with the two food challenges, converting one or both to OIT if Alex didn't pass.

The food challenge was an individualized portion of Alex's OIT journey. The beauty and success of OIT is that it takes a basic protocol and tailors it to each patient and their bodies specific allergens and challenges during the process. Our allergist was simply choosing to do an "ingestion" to monitor what happened and see if OIT was necessary before the months of trips and the years of daily maintenance ingestion ahead of him. He had reasons and research behind this step. I want to be clear that not everyone's OIT journey starts or includes a food challenge or challenges at the beginning, but Alex's did.

We set up the magic day, April 14th. In about three weeks, it would begin. For sanity's sake, I made the first appointment, and then tucked that away on the calendar as something that was happening later. I needed to keep being present in life for my kids now, not trembling in the future with incessant online research.

Since I had tabled my anxiety about the appointment, the night before our departure, it floated immediately up to the surface. Four hours in the car as a passenger with everyone occupied got my head spinning, my fingers typing, and my heart racing. I had chosen to take Alex, and he was willing, to an appointment to food challenge walnuts and peanuts, and I was terrified.

To choose to have him eat something that I knew he was allergic to suddenly, sitting in that car rather than thinking about it in the allergist's office, seemed liked willful harm. I had to find a way to calm myself down before we were out of the car and Alex could see my distress. I needed to be a calm parent at his side. I wasn't as worried about the walnut as he had eaten walnuts for 10 of his 16 years until that one incident in South Dakota. Plus, his current walnut labs were showing zero and the skin test had been negative. Plus, he'd only had a skin test at our original allergist, never lab work. I knew now the inaccuracy of his original walnut allergy testing.

But those peanuts, they had me spiraling down into all sorts of disaster rabbit holes. My head rationally and logically had found all the research to calm me down and see the safety and wisdom of pursuing OIT, but I hadn't gotten my teeth into the actual protocol of a food challenge. I hadn't researched food challenges enough, and I was fearful. The allergist had explained them that day, but I hadn't researched them prior or since then.

Luckily, while researching in the car, I found reliable sources to address and quiet exactly what I was worried about. One, from a reliable food allergy group, detailed how food challenge was the "gold standard" of diagnosis as the allergist had told us. Reading about the actual specifics of a food challenge and what it entailed versus what I thought from my experience of Alex accidentally ingesting peanuts was eye opening.

He wasn't going in the morning to sit down and eat a peanut. It would be minute amounts in solution over a period of time to safely see if he would start to react. If he did, it would stop immediately. He would be monitored for breathing and blood pressure and pulse the entire time. He would be cognizant and old enough to describe and communicate what he was feeling physically and emotionally.

In my self-talk, I reasoned Alex would have an accidental ingestion again one day; it could be a week, it could be years, but statistically and historically, I knew he would have an ingestion. He'd already had five with parents and loved ones that knew everything to do and look for. We were simply choosing to give more knowledge to his allergy by doing that ingesting while we had close medical monitoring.

The other thing that I learned is that Alex mostly fears the *Epipen* injector in the event of an accidental ingestion and if the food challenge failed. Have you ever witnessed how an *Epipen* injects? It is basically a forceful needle rocket. This is so that it goes deep into the muscle tissue for those inexperienced with a needle. It also needs to be able to go through clothing. Well, in a food challenge this is not how epinephrine would be administered by our allergist. Instead, if needed, it would be administered delicately and gently like a shot, using a smaller more comfortable needle, not the large injector rocket needle.

Also, since he would be in a medically supervised setting with monitoring, the epinephrine was more of a last resort. There were protocols in place to ensure if the monitoring didn't pick up a systemic or several system reaction going on, the food challenge would be halted. At the first sign of throat bothering or stomach upset, the peanut solution would be stopped and Alex would be given meds to comfort the symptom he developed.

There was time and notice due to the slow individualized protocol before Alex would ever approach a situation like the anaphylactic reactions he had previously, outside of a doctor's office, which resulted in an epinephrine injection. I also found an article about the levels of lab results in the peanut component panel. I made a note to ask the allergist before starting the food challenge to explain in greater detail Alex's combination of proteins and their numbers in relation to how the markers linked to anaphylaxis.

At the end of the four hour drive, I had convinced the fear monster inside of me again that a food challenge was the next best step in taking action to see if OIT could save Alex from a life of avoidance and fear. One controlled possible reaction with an expert doctor was a positive decision and a step towards making Alex safer. I wasn't putting him in harm's way; I was helping him walk one step farther from harm's way. I kept repeating in my head: Love not fear, hope not fear.

I hugged Alex that night and told him I was proud of his bravery and shared that I knew he probably picked up on my anxiety, but that I felt in my head and my heart that this was the best step to take. It was a step that made him safer. I acknowledged that I imagined it was scary to eat his allergens willfully for the first time tomorrow morning. We joked that he knew he could certainly do it calmer than worry wart me.

He shared with me that he had convinced himself that he might not be allergic, so tomorrow when he ate walnut or peanut, he was going to stay calm. He would remember the lack of a skin test reaction last month, the charts that the allergist had shown us of his labs versus others in OIT and different ages of life. "Plus," Alex told me matter of factly, "This is a necessary thing to rule out before beginning; it's just like another test or lab." His calmness amazed me. He was glad to hear that it wasn't an *Epipen* injector, but instead a gentle needle that awaited him if he started to react during the food challenge and needed epinephrine. He said he could handle a shot; it was those injectors that were stress inducing.

Walnut Challenge

We planned for the challenge to be a daylong event. One food challenge in the morning, and if that went well, then one in the afternoon. We got ushered into a room with all our materials for chilling for the day, iPad's, iPhones, books, and a guitar. We had a good, but light breakfast with some protein so Alex would not have an empty stomach. He'd been taking probiotics and another vitamin for several weeks that were a part of this allergist's protocol.

Alex was ready. I asked my final question about the specifics of peanut component labs. And as the doctor explained, I began to feel calmer. It wouldn't be that different from starting OIT. He would either have to stop at a certain point, which would decide the much lower starting OIT dose, or he would continue to slowly receive more allergen if the doctor didn't see any signs of Alex reacting, which would indicate he had passed.

Alex and Dr. A chose together to do the walnut challenge first. I don't know what walnut OIT protocols are, but Alex's food challenge started with some tiny particles of actual walnut. They looked like sawdust, just a few flecks. He was to take them and drink a good bit of water. Then every 15 minutes or so more particles were taken in increasing amounts. None of the walnut doses did anything to Alex. He had no reaction whatsoever.

By the time the morning was over, Alex tolerated eating two walnuts out of a cup. He said that walnuts had a bland taste, but he survived eating them. He passed his walnut food challenge! The added fear of accidentally eating walnut based on his bread reaction and skin tests that we had carried for five years was gone. Just like that, in four hours.

No more worrying about pesto. No more avoiding the homemade brownies someone added walnuts to. No more worrying about the walnut trees growing everywhere where we live. Whatever walnut or otherwise that had caused his reaction and his resulting positive skin test in 2012 was either gone or was never valid to begin with. Since our local allergist had not suggested blood work for the walnut, feeling the skin prick, large welt, and reaction to the banana bread were enough for a diagnosis, we had no way to know if anything had been a false positive back then.

We could have walnuts back in our house. We could stop being afraid of all the paleo diet items that were popping up–as they often had walnuts as a flour or a nut milk in them. This was such a celebratory feeling, to take walnut off the food avoidance list. I practically skipped out of the office to go and get some lunch; I was elated.

Alex was supposed to eat carbs at lunch to keep his body in the best state for eating allergens. There are a lot of tricks and science to back up protocols in OIT to make dosing and eating an allergen acclimate best in the body. Carbohydrates and apples are common foods consumed with an OIT dose. I don't remember the specifics of carbs. As for apples, this fruit and applesauce or other derivatives of apples are used by some OIT allergists as a part of the dosing protocol. This is due to the polyphenols in apple that somehow help mediate the allergen in the body.

I drank wine to celebrate, and honestly, to help calm me down a bit for the peanut eating afternoon that lay ahead. As Alex left the table to use the bathroom, I burst into tears. I couldn't expect a fear I held and saw in action for 16 years disappear all because of some lowered blood tests, a negative skin test, and an expert allergist's opinion. Since Alex hadn't had a reaction to peanuts yet as a teen, I did worry that this ingestion, this controlled planned purposeful ingestion of peanut, would be different and more severe and scarier than before.

I feared it would be like every teen death from peanut ingestion that I had ever read about, and I'd be sitting right there while it happened having chosen and convinced my son to try it. This was completely illogical because no patient has ever died doing an OIT food challenge or protocol. But it was in my head, a product of the fear and anxiety I carried around. All my logical rationalizing and reading during the drive over that had calmed my nerves was slipping away as the hour he would eat peanut approached. I'd slipped back into terror.

Kurt confirmed that he too was afraid, but he knew and still felt it was the right thing to do. The office food challenge was safer than any reaction Alex had before or would ever have in his future life have again. He said we needed to be strong and carry on. I concurred and handed a little more of the responsibility to Kurt and Alex for this day and this peanut challenge that was about to happen. I collected my tears before Alex came back to the table. I didn't want to add anything to the weight he was carrying.

I had the urge to say a prayer, but I didn't know what to say. I have a myriad of ways to pause for help or to physically move through emotions and hard times full of grief and loss, but prayer isn't one of my normal tools. I admire, respect, and honor the facets of all world religions that give ritual and intentional moments to our human lives that are filled with fear and scary and unknown moments. I understand the human need to have a physical place and structure to place ourselves to deal with the reality of the world and have community. I was needing a place like that right now to put myself in to have faith and peace.

I promptly went to the parking lot and called my dear Catholic friend and told her that I needed a saint and a prayer to say over Alex for his impending ingestion of peanuts, so that I could calm down, even though I wasn't Catholic. If there would have been a labyrinth nearby, I could have walked my fear in, set it down physically by leaving a trinket and walked out more peaceful. If I were more experienced at meditation, I could have perhaps gotten to a Zen place with a sit down or a walk around. I didn't have time nor these tools at my disposal. If I'd had a Xanax prescription, I'd have taken one. I didn't have a way to set down this fear. I needed to mark the setting down some way so I could walk back into that allergy office and watch Alex ingest peanut. Knowing all the science of OIT and the food challenge did nothing to shut off or ignore the fear of Alex eating peanuts.

I needed a divine intervention. My friend delivered. She gave me a Saint, complete with the words to recite for Alex. As we drove back to the allergist's, I asked Alex if he would humor his mom and let me say a prayer with him. I acknowledged it was out of the ordinary for me, but I felt so helpless in the task of setting the fear and responsibility down that I had to do something. If I had it all wrong and there was a God looking down on me in disapproval for allowing Alex to go through this, I wanted a Hail Mary. I wanted Alex to be given mercy. He rolled his eyes and obliged me. There by his side in the car, I laid my hand on him and recited my plea to the Saint of the day. Catholic for an afternoon worked to calm me down and allow whatever was going to happen to begin.

CHAPTER 12 - STARTING PEANUT OIT

We arrived back at the office to start the peanut food challenge. It was a different process than the walnut challenge. I came in from that emotional lunch elated Alex had passed walnut and hopeful he would pass peanut, but I was skeptical.

When the nurse asked us how we were doing upon our return to the office, I jokingly asked if she had any anxiety medications to dose the parents. She laughed and I imagine wasn't quite sure what to do with me. I'm not sure she had seen anyone as anxious as me. I'd seen my kid eat something with peanut in it and react five times. I don't know how many older patients they see with parents who have given their kid an epinephrine injector five times. The nurse and allergist saw kids eat their allergen all the time, so no fear or trepidation radiated from them, only calm.

The allergist advised that peanuts were going to be different than the walnut challenge. Each food was a bit different than another in how the allergen was introduced and dosed, due to the potency, the oils, and how bodies seemed to respond; peanut was a lot slower and would be in a solution starting at a minuscule amount, building up to 3mg, less than one percent of a peanut. This is part of the beauty of OIT: it is individualized for each patient from protocols developed in research trials and by pioneering allergists who started training others on the protocols over the past decade.

Alex said he was good to go, so after checking his vitals and readying his mind, he took his first dose of peanut. It was a syringe of mostly clear looking solution that looked like the type of dispenser you would give a toddler liquid medicine in. Alex took the dose and said that it tasted smoky. Probably any description he gave would send me into full body tension, but smoky definitely did because smoky was close to spicy.

I told him that was interesting and succeeded at not conveying any anxiety to Alex. Alex already felt nervous, worried his concern over eating peanut would somehow lead to a false positive reaction. The doctor had assured him that he was calm, and he wasn't going to cause a false positive reaction. Alex would know if he didn't feel great, and if he had body systems react, then it was real as he couldn't make his body react systemically just by thinking of it.

It was surreal. My grown up first baby, taller than me and the allergist, sat on a chair on a path to eating peanuts safely. He calmly played the latest massively multiplayer online game of the week on the iPad he had brought. He nonchalantly sat there emanating typical teen indifference to what was going on around him. I sat in the chair nearby texting family and siblings at home that were anxious to know what was happening.

Kurt and I were exchanging knowing fearful, hopeful eyes and big blinks at each other across the room. I think that I got through that first 15-20 minutes of the first dose with only asking Alex once as uninterested as I could, which I think was good acting, "How are you doing?"

"Hmm," eyes not coming up from his screen, "just fine," he answered. He was calm, chill, and relaxed. Like he would be any other afternoon at home.

Alex went up in minute doses every 15-20 minutes. Nothing changed for Alex with any of these additions of solution. He played his game, talked with us intermittently, sipped his water, made eye contact, and didn't feel worried. Then he got to the fourth syringe of solution, which equaled roughly double the typical OIT starting dose. The usual starting OIT peanut dose for the majority of patients is 3mg, about 1% of a peanut, which is a tolerance level that 95% of patients can ingest in the beginning without a reaction (OIT101, 2016d).

About a minute or two in after this fourth syringe, Alex's energy changed. He shifted in the chair he was in and got up. There was a brief pace across the small room, and then he was sitting on the exam table. I held back asking if anything was wrong while everything in me was screaming at the visual clues his body was giving.

He had stopped a clue based game he was engaged in for no reason other than to go sit on the table. Before I had the chance to ask my question, he piped up. "Mom, my ribs feel tight, like in my chest." We called the allergist in to alert him and get closer monitoring. Alex described the feeling in his chest like a slight pressure, and an itchy throat. All his vitals stayed level, no hives, no other mouth, oral, breathing, or gastrointestinal symptoms happened.

Then there was one more syringe of solution. After a period, the itchy throat and chest pressure had subsided. After that last dose, Alex expressed that his stomach felt slightly upset, like a gnawing feeling, the beginning feeling if you were to get hungry, dizzy, or nauseous. The pacing along with these two mild symptoms that had replaced his interest in his game were noticeable.

The allergist called off the food challenge right then and there and halted the stomach symptom with medication, not epinephrine as it wasn't an anaphylactic reaction. Alex didn't get any worse and felt better in about five to ten minutes. The allergist said that Alex's change in demeanor along with two of his systems having mild discomfort at different doses, no matter how mild, meant that progressing to more peanut would be likely to produce a reaction that would escalate to anaphylaxis based on Alex's labs and lifelong history.

It was enough to know that he had gotten this far. The food challenge confirmed that he did in fact still react to peanut even with lower labs and a negative skin test at age sixteen. We now knew definitively that spending time, money, effort, and travel to complete this OIT process was necessary and valid for us and Alex. His OIT journey began that moment as we were sent home with a daily dose of slightly more than the standard starting dose for peanut, Alex's daily dose was about half the amount he had gotten to before stopping his food challenge.

I was relieved that the peanut challenge was over. I was disappointed it had ended differently than the walnut, but also glad it had been uneventful and given us the data we needed. I was grateful that all that failing of a food challenge entailed was a bit of solution, some mild discomfort, and a handful of meds. As we sat there for the further hours of monitoring before Alex was released, the grief set in.

This grief is something that I would have never planned on or expected. For me, these two hours after the failed peanut food challenge ended up being the hardest two hours of the whole OIT process. My son had been allergic to peanuts his whole eating life, why was this such a defeated feeling like I was just finding out? Mostly it was an empathetic response to what I saw Alex lying there feeling. A toxic cocktail of emotions.

A part of him worried he had indeed psyched himself into a reaction by having a panic attack. But, the allergist talked him out of that self-blaming idea, explaining that the symptoms he was having were real, and that it wasn't something he could have caused by thinking them into being. But another part of him was devastated like it was the first time he learned he was allergic to peanuts. Alex had done such an excellent job convincing himself he wasn't allergic in order to enter this food challenge day full of confidence and without anxiety; thus, it was like he was finding out at age 16 that he had a life-threatening peanut allergy.

Since he had been allergic and avoiding peanuts before age two, he had no conscious memory of finding out his allergy news fresh and feeling that sentence of scarcity. He had always lived in a peanut avoiding and peanut free world. Embarking on this OIT journey and wrapping his head and heart around the idea of not being allergic and the possibility of having outgrown the severity of his allergy had grown on him. He had lived for three weeks with that abundant hopeful feeling that he had never experienced. It was crushing to have it whisked out from under him like a rug. It left him a bruised mess there in the office for a while.

I think this emotional reaction worried the doctor. So, I had to explain what was going on: it wasn't a further physical reaction, it was an emotional disappointment. I could glimpse it but I couldn't understand it; I could only imagine the feeling. The allergist probably couldn't understand that grief either because he knew that there would be OIT success at the end of this. This sadness was an aspect of a failed food challenge that I hadn't expected.

We didn't have the hindsight the allergist had. All we knew was Alex had mustered up every ounce of bravery that he had and several milliliters of a smoky bean liquid had drowned it within an hour. He needed to grieve. And so, we did. I just hugged him, or didn't hug him as the moment warranted. As his mom, I sat there for that hour and a half second guessing every choice I had made regarding exploring OIT.

Here I had an emotionally healthy teen that had learned to be empowered and live confidently and abundantly, mostly without restrictions, with his allergy, and here I'd gone and undone all the good mental health we had built up about it.

A myriad of questions bounced around in my brain: Was OIT going to be worth it? Was Alex going to regress in his confidence and life living with allergy? Was he more scared in OIT than he'd been before? Should I be relieved if he were a little more scared because it made him safer to be scared? What did that say about me if I was? What kind of mother wants their child to be afraid? What if it made it worse for him? What kind of mother weighs and sacrifices her autonomous teen son's mental health and physical health to put him in a safer path so that she feels less responsible as he grows older? Who was I to make that decision? Had I manipulated him into trying this? Were my motives all pure? Was I attempting to shut off my guilty ego for having contributed to this allergy in some way by what I ate when I was pregnant, by heredity, by breastfeeding him as I ate peanuts? Was my need to rectify that guilt, to try and undo it by finding a food allergy treatment for the emotional baggage of food avoidance selfish? Had I put him in a spot where he was feeling more trauma than he had as a young kid for any of the right reasons? I was sinking into feelings of self-doubt, wondering if I was selfish, sitting there waiting to be in the clear reaction time to leave for home.

This was the roller coaster moment during OIT that I didn't know would hit me. I imagine for every parent and kid it would be different to sit there and fail a food challenge. For some, it would be no big deal. But it hit me big, and it hit Alex that day. It didn't hit me hard enough to back out of pursuing OIT because I had physically seen Alex ingest a small amount of peanut protein and NOT have an anaphylactic reaction. He did have a threshold, and that threshold could be increased as he became desensitized.

If anything, I now trusted OIT more, seeing it in reality rather than simply on paper and screens. It was just the regret at losing the hope he had outgrown it; at not getting him into a trial ten years ago; that as a mom, I couldn't protect him from this pain of finding out basically anew of his allergy at 16.

Alex was holding his allergy as his more than ever before. He was the one allergic to the peanut, and he was doing this treatment to live safer with that reality. I was here to cheer, to drive him back and forth, and to be his sounding board. Having lived a life full of striving to avoid food struggle, it was painful to have chosen to cause it at this food challenge appointment.

We left the doctor's office that April day, but not without looking back, because that's all we did on the drive home and until the next day. We looked back at what we'd lived through and what lay ahead. I realized the confidence this gave me to do OIT for Alex. I saw that it was needed and that every painful part of it would be valuable because it was baby steps away from fear. I would never wonder if he would have maybe outgrown his allergy or made it to ingestion one day without OIT. We'd know now that it was for sure the OIT that got him there.

Back at home, it seemed that after the drive and a full night's sleep, we had finished processing. I started our next day in planning mode. Alex didn't balk. I planned to be OIT dose ready. I researched ways and products and methods to hold his dose if he had an event away from home for the day. I didn't want dosing daily to feel like he was being held back.

There was a pack used for insulin that would keep a bit of solution cool enough to not spoil if his busy teen day had him away from the fridge at dosing time. We could still go on the camping trip with our friends that was coming up. I was primed to deal with this as creatively and confidently as I could. We hadn't done anything but carry *EpiPens*, keeping them at the right temperature, for years so these months of being married to a refrigerated solution until Alex was on actual peanut pieces were a challenge. I'm not going to lie, for a good few weeks, it felt like a burden to have to take this refrigerated solution every day at a certain time.

We hadn't felt like we were carrying a physical burden that kept us from going and doing for so long. All our food allergy avoidance burdens were emotional at this point in his life. I did think a few times, had I thought this through? Before OIT, he was quite free to come and go as he pleased if he had his *EpiPen*. Does OIT make him freer because now he must dose in this window of time and rest in this window of time and carry this other stuff with him that can't fit in a pocket?

At first I got a little irritated at this, but then I chose to reframe it. This was a brief time frame in his life, a tradeoff for so much more. This was silly and privileged of me to feel irritated at something that was not that complicated. It wasn't a lifetime of injections; it wasn't a life-saving burden of medicating some condition and the expense and the fear that would come with that. It was a life-giving opportunity to get to the normal side of life that parents and kids around us had been living for sixteen years.

I wanted to feel normal. I wanted to not worry. I wanted to be free of the fear and anxiety. I committed to positively play the OIT game and get Alex through this portion of refrigerated dosing that seemed like a step backwards.

CHAPTER 13 - UPDOSING APPOINTMENTS

A fter the food challenge appointment on April 14, 2016, Alex had sixteen more updose appointments until he reached peanut "maintenance mode" on December 28, 2016. (Updosing is when you go in after a period of time, in our case it was about every two weeks, to get a new slightly higher daily dose.) Over that time, Alex went from ingesting less than .003 grams of peanut, about 1% of a peanut, to eating 7 grams, about 7-8 peanuts, daily. He will hold at that for a year or more, where he will then have more labs done, and the opportunity to do another peanut food challenge.

If he passes that larger food challenge amount and his labs have done what they are supposed to, Alex could graduate to being able to "free eat" peanuts in his diet beyond his daily dose. We traveled eighteen times including the consult to the allergy office in a neighboring state to do OIT with Alex. Each visit for us was a three and a half to four-hour trip one way. We drove over 3,300 miles in those eight months getting Alex this amazing food allergy treatment.

Each updose visit was about two weeks apart, some were a little farther apart if we had a conflict that kept us from traveling back to the office sooner. A few visits were a little closer than that. The OIT doctor wouldn't do updose appointments closer than ten days apart. So, Alex had a few visits that were ten days apart when we had larger gaps coming up due to a trip or another conflict. We went early those times because it would be better to get in sooner rather than later to avoid getting off a progressing schedule.

For about the first three months of the updosing appointments, we arranged to drive over the night before and stay in a nearby hotel. The remaining five months were primarily one of us driving Alex there and back in one day, having a midday or just before lunch appointment and then coming home. We also dealt with a time change getting to our updose appointment. So, that three and a half to four-hour trip was in effect closer to five hours on one end.

One time my aunt, Alex's great aunt, at the energetic and adventurous age of 75 drove with Alex to his appointment when Kurt and I both had a conflict. Instead of rescheduling the appointment, it was a great gift to have her offer to drive him. This arrangement was approved in advance by the allergist.

Over the eight months that Alex was in OIT, we usually left our other children at home. There were exceptions to this. One time we did updosing on the way home from camp, and everyone came along because there was a vacation on the other side of that visit. Another time, we drove a few extra hours the day before on our way out of town for a homeschool field trip at Dauphin Island Sea Lab to do the updosing appointment in route to the field trip.

The times we had to make an OIT appointment into a two-day affair, we made it an overnight that we wanted to be there for. One overnight trip we visited a store we had always wanted to see. Another overnight we saw fabulous art exhibits by Vik Munoz and Eric Carle, and we got to explore the DeKalb Farmers Market like we hadn't since the kids were little for a whole afternoon. We used rewards programs and points and stayed in hotels with included breakfast buffets. When we said yes to the OIT appointment that had to be an overnight, we said yes to making it a memory and a part of our learning. Friends came with Alex to OIT two different times, once on the visit on the way home from camp and once on the visit on the way to the sea lab field trip.

Overall, we spent one hundred and forty-four hours traveling in the car to get Alex into the office for his updosing appointments. I once jokingly changed the lyrics of the song, "I'm Gonna Be (500 miles)" made famous in the movie *Benny & Joon* to *"But I would drive 200 miles, And I would drive 200 more, Just to be the mom who drove 400 hundred miles, To OIT at your door!"* I sang it loud and glad happily driving to the allergist's doorstep.

We tried to break up the monotony of traveling to OIT by adding in outings, including outings with friends. One time in the summer we tacked on a day at the aquarium following an early morning OIT appointment with some friends who drove over that morning. After one OIT visit upon being cleared for eating at places with open shelled peanuts such as Five Guys, we celebrated by driving home through Chattanooga and meeting friends there for art space exploring, downtown walking, and the highlight of the night, a dinner with a crowd of friends for the first time at Five Guys!

We tried to make OIT updosing a normal part of life, as normal as driving eight hours in a day every two weeks in a family of six can be. We also tried to make it as special as possible. In the OIT community, it is a desired outcome that OIT be boring because if OIT is boring, that means that everything is just clipping right along with no bumps in the road. Alex's OIT journey was boring.

Even though it was eight months and so much driving and traveling, it seemed to zoom by. Everyone's OIT protocol is tailored directly to them and their reaction history and their goals to be bite safe or free eating safe, so I don't share these details to imply that this is what another person's journey would look like. This is just what Alex's journey from start to finish looked like, and from my time on the OIT groups, it's a pretty normal looking journey. A progression of updoses for his allergen over months or a year's time culminating in graduation to maintenance.

Eating Peanut Pieces

Three months into OIT, Alex's dose changed from solution to actual peanut pieces. The peanut pieces were such tiny fragments in the cup, but they did look more ominous than the cloudy solution he had been taking.

He took the dose of peanut fragments without a problem. I was giddy at the reality of this. He had technically been eating peanuts for months, but it still felt like a medicine when it was in solution form, like a magic potion he was taking each day. These bits in this plastic medicine cup were just peanuts. The same as those peanut food pieces I had visualized and could spot anywhere for 16 years.

This was the moment in OIT for me where the wolf came out of the sheep's clothing. Peanut had been hiding, looking safe and innocuous in that cloudy solution Alex had been squirting in his mouth every day. Here it was uncloaked, undiluted, just pieces of nuts in a cup. That night after we drove back home from this updosing, I headed to the store to buy peanuts.

I hadn't bought peanuts in over 15 years! Once we had become to a nut free household when Alex was two, I had never shopped again for a peanut or a jar of peanut butter. I will admit on the occasional trip away from the kids, I did eat a few peanut butter cups over the years, but grocery shopping for peanuts, never! I had done my research as to what types to buy to replicate what the doctor wanted him to have. I headed in shopping for dry, unsalted roasted peanuts. This form had the right oil and water and protein makeup to match the milligram dosage that Alex was on.

Publix carried the Hampton Farms brand peanuts in the shell. I bought them as they were on a lot of parent and doctor recommended lists. We didn't have to worry about cross contamination with tree nuts like some OIT patients do, but I wanted to get peanuts that others were using. It felt like I was buying illicit drugs at the checkout counter, or venomous snakes. My brain was screaming. They let you sell these in here? Am I really buying these peanuts? It was like buying alcohol legally for the first time when I turned twenty-one.

Then while driving away, I started to think about how to get these peanuts in the shell in dosage form; we would need to remove the shells and deal with the dust and mess. How could Alex measure his own doses if he had to shell peanuts? Could he shell peanuts? I didn't know if other teens doing OIT had their parents shell the nuts, or if they used already shelled peanuts. I turned away from home to head to Whole Foods, thinking surely they would have some shelled, dry roasted, unsalted nuts. They did have a store brand, 365 Degrees, bag of roasted, unsalted peanuts, and again I did the unthinkable. I bought peanuts in broad daylight to take to my house to dose my peanut allergic child.

When Alex's dose went from solution to peanut pieces, the reality of the freedom of OIT first started to set in. I was going to have the allergen that could cause anaphylaxis in the house again; he was going to eat it every day. The peanut's threat and control over our lives was on the way out. As Alex was becoming desensitized to the peanut, the peanut was sensitizing me to see it as only the bean that it was.

Odd Moments in the Dosing Journey

I mentioned before the idea of OIT being boring as a good thing. While I said his journey wasn't boring in the sense that we enjoyed the travel, Alex's journey was boring in that it went without incident. Some patients complete OIT without having completely boring journeys. Private practice OIT allergists are heroes, and the OIT process can be designed to progress as slow or as fast as the allergy will allow. It is not a race.

This is what makes OIT an individualized treatment. There are ways to get through the rough patches and finish the protocol in the majority of cases. However, Alex had no speed bumps on his OIT road. That is to say that he never down dosed (had to alter a dose due to a reaction) or stopped dosing (had to stop and start OIT at another point due to a reaction). The only two hiccups that dotted his map were completely random and out of the blue. These two moments stood out but they never approached the level of an anaphylactic reaction or a near miss. They were just odd incidents that happened twice during the eight months of his OIT protocol. OIT desensitizes the immune system and the gastrointestinal system, and sometimes, there is stomach discomfort.

His first odd moment came in the summer about four months in. Alex was dosing in the afternoon at this point. He had been with us at my parents' house for most of the day. He had taken his dose like normal, on a full stomach, snacking with applesauce and plenty of water, and rested afterwards for the allotted time. In order to get home early that evening, he decided to scooter back home on a foot powered manual scooter that was at my parents' house.

Alex is a very active teen: he skateboards on a long board he built, does CrossFit, swims, runs occasionally, and played Ultimate

Frisbee in a summer league last year. So, scootering the mile it took to get home from my parents' was no big deal to him, just some wind in his hair. After he got home, he called me. "Mom," he said, "I don't know why, but my chest feels tight after scootering; it's that tight feeling like when I first did the peanut food challenge."

I told him to take his prescribed antihistamine, and I'd call the doctor and be right there. We got the allergist on the phone; he assessed how Alex was feeling otherwise, and since the tight chest feeling hadn't lingered other than a short few minutes and had gone away immediately upon rest and meds, he advised that there was nothing else to do than be alert for any other symptoms. He did recommend an antacid for Alex instead of antihistamine if that feeling came again on another day as it sounded more like heartburn. Alex dosed the next day, and that tight chest feeling never returned.

I was left not knowing if it was just a chest pain from scootering or a real OIT related symptom from his daily dose that had happened hours earlier. What I did realize, which gave me a big relief, was seeing how aware and in-tune Alex was to his body. He had experienced an odd feeling, and he could immediately go into the mindset of caution. He had quickly identified that this feeling he had might be related to his dose, and he had called me to get the doctor involved. This slight chest pain was minimal compared to the starting symptoms of reactions he had had prior to OIT, and yet he was still able, even though it was minor, to immediately give it serious and respectful attention.

This again confirmed that OIT was the right thing for Alex. OIT wasn't giving him false security; it was just giving him a larger safety net and other safety ropes to grab onto. He was just as aware of watching his body for a peanut anaphylaxis reaction as he had been before. Honestly, I think he was more aware. He had that many more experiences of eating his allergen beyond the five ingestions prior to when he turned 16 and started OIT.

He had been eating peanut in small amount for four months, 120 days since his food challenge in April. Every day he dosed, he was learning about eating his allergen. He was aware of when the taste changed from smoky to tasting like beans to neutral or not bad. OIT gave him authentic, in-tune, empowering safety. We no longer had to live based in fear, waiting to see when the reaction would appear.

The second odd moment happened in route to Austin, Texas, to visit my sister, six months in to OIT. We were on one of those long car rides that takes two days to complete. The car was full with all four kids; me; and our dog, Oliver. In order to get out the door faster, we stopped for breakfast on the road instead of spending time and mess eating at home. These days in OIT, Alex was cleared to eat items that might have cross contamination as well as peanut oil again due to the dosage level he was at. We were always excited to do the things that had a ban lifted on them, so I encouraged taking those new steps.

Alex had not eaten at Chick-Fil-A since he was a toddler. Even though the refined peanut oil is reported to not have proteins and to not affect those that are allergic, we had experienced pinprick type hives on Alex's mouth when he ate Chick-Fil-A. We had phased it out of his and our eating plan to be on the safe side and to create as little reaction and inflammation in his body as possible. It didn't matter that experts said peanut oil wasn't allergic, Alex didn't consume it.

Since being cleared for peanut oil and cross contamination labeled foods, Chick-Fil-A had been back on our menu. So far Alex had only had the fries, which in truth aren't fried in peanut oil anymore anyway, but that was what he wanted and felt safe eating there to start. That morning, Alex decided to try the chicken breakfast sandwich. I was excited for him. I had lived a big part of my working life prior to his birth eating one of these every day for breakfast, as there was a Chick-Fil-A in the parking lot of the place I worked in those years. I was excited for my kid, who loved to eat, to enjoy the greasy and flaky goodness of a Chick-Fil-A biscuit. I even encouraged him to try it with some jelly on it. He enjoyed it. Nothing out of sorts happened after breakfast was over.

Six or eight hours later in our day of traveling, we stopped at rest areas; ran some sprints; ate some snacks; had lunch; and enjoyed a lovely dog park in Monroe, LA, with Oliver. We had just finished eating an early dinner while it was still daylight sitting outside on the pet patio at Jason's Deli, and afterwards, Alex had taken his OIT dose.

Within about 20 minutes, Alex said he felt weird. First his throat had an irritated feeling, but by the time we had the doctor on the phone, that had stopped but his stomach felt uneasy, kind of nauseous. We hadn't left the exit we were at, and I had already located the nearest ER, administered the antihistamine and antacid that the doctor recommended and got Alex some more applesauce and water from inside the drugstore we had pulled over at.

This feeling could have been due to the food he'd just eaten, maybe some cross contamination of his sandwich at Jason's Deli, combined with his dose. The peanut dose on top of the first Chick-Fil-A sandwich that morning worried me. The allergist assured me that there was likely not a causality to the discomfort at dosing and the peanut oil. He said this just sometimes happens due to the gastrointestinal system adjusting. Maybe traveling all day factored in to it; it could be any number of things disrupting his normal dose experience.

Within minutes of the apples and medicine, all stomach discomfort was gone and the throat feeling that had migrated to the stomach never returned. We were good to keep traveling and proceed without concern after waiting a period. We drove on to our hotel for the night and enjoyed the rest of our trip to Austin, including a camping trip with friends on the way back home, without any further odd incidents.

CHAPTER 14 - TRAVELING

Traveling *WITH OIT*

Like anything new, the first few weeks of OIT dosing seemed like a sudden complication to a life that we had become familiar with. Spontaneity was common in our days, and as long as we packed the *EpiPen* in our bags and held in our fear, we headed out of the house on a whim. Initially, it felt constricting that the dose needed to be refrigerated, Alex had to consume the dose in a certain window, and he had to rest for a period of time after dosing.

The daily required medication seemed daunting to a mom and kid who hadn't dealt with that before. Keeping Alex safe by avoiding peanuts was a different sort of daunting every day; it was more chaotic than scheduled. I was used to tacking a mental safety checklist onto any outing or moment, but I wasn't skilled at adding on a physical daily habit. We weren't used to many daily habits other than eating, sleeping, brushing our teeth, and focusing on learning and peace at home. Because of the freedom inherent in the way we had chosen to learn, we did not have a structured day to day school schedule and instead let each day's path and learning flow from the interests and experiences of the one before. This meant that many a day looked different than the one before. Fitting a daily OIT dose reliably into this environment took some creative thinking.

I kind of panicked in these first few weeks, wondering how we could have any more of the adventure filled days of learning we had crafted for the past 11 years now that we were tied to a dose every day. I put on my creative hat and became determined to twist the rules, to bend the protocols outside of what it said on the paper. If the dose was refrigerated, taken within the window of dosing time, and there was rest and observation on hand, then we would still do whatever we needed or wanted to do.

I asked questions in groups and found that most people didn't travel as much with their early doses as I wanted to. Many probably were not used to frequent travel either because they were on school/work schedules that were more static, or they just didn't desire to, or they didn't have the means to have day trips nearby their home. Some families were using insulin cooling travel cases to hold a dose for travel. That was so bulky, and again I wanted Alex to have no qualms over having to carry more than just an *EpiPen* with him. I didn't want him to have to carry a bigger bag. To solve this, I found a small, Yeti-type beverage container with a screw on lid. It fit in his messenger bag or backpack just like a small water bottle and could hold his solution bottle and syringe for dosing.

In those first months, if we were headed out for the day, that OIT solution got measured into a bottle and went inside the beverage cooler I kept at the ready in the freezer with ice chilled inside the bottom of it. For a longer car trip, we took a bottle of peanut flour/powder (that our allergist gave us at each updose if we asked as a spare) that didn't have the water added to it yet so that it could stay shelf stable until we were at our destination. Once there, we could add water to it and then refrigerate it.

I could have taken an eight-month hiatus from normal life to make OIT dosing easier, and I would have, but I was doing this to get more out of life for Alex. I knew if he were going to buy into it for the long term as a teen and young adult, it had to be done in a way that didn't stop or interfere with the freedom and full life he had already built.

We didn't let OIT dosing define our day; we did give it reverence and honored the protocol, but we inserted it creatively into every day that wasn't a day at home. There wasn't a day or event that we ever had to cancel during Alex's OIT journey. OIT could be successfully added to a busy teen's life. He had one day he missed dosing completely later in his OIT journey, and so he did a "split dose" (halving his dose and taking it in two batches twenty minutes apart) the following day to get back on track. The doctor assured us that occasionally in OIT a dosing day is missed due to illness or other circumstances. Under the supervision of the allergist, the process has protocols to account for that and to get the patient back on the daily dose the next day safely. In Alex's case and the point he was at, that meant splitting his dose for one day.

You can travel extensively while doing Oral Immunotherapy once you have the dosing time, protocol, and allergen storage figured out. I already shared the miles and hours of travel for actual OIT updose appointments that we logged. Along with that, Alex also experienced other completely unrelated travel in the eight months he was doing OIT to get to his maintenance dose level.

OIT doesn't have to stop a child, teen, or adult's traveling. Here are all the spots Alex traveled to over the eight months he was doing OIT. It's a long list. You can travel to do OIT, and you can travel while you do OIT!

To Decatur, AL, for a soccer tournament with friends visiting from Louisiana.

To Birmingham, AL, on a tour of the Golden Flake snack food's company.

To attend a weekend backpacking trip at a remote rustic wilderness lodge, Charit Creek Lodge, located in Big South Fork National Recreation Area in northern Tennessee.

To Springville, AL, to compete in the Panther Run, a mudslinging obstacle course.

To go tent camping at a state park in north Georgia with his aunt and two other families to visit Howard Finster's Paradise Gardens.

To Lynchburg, TN, to celebrate his great-aunt's 75th birthday with a meal at Miss Mary Bobo's Boarding House Restaurant.

To Memphis, TN, for three days to visit friends that were there from Washington State.

To Grayton Beach, FL, for a week for our 58th family reunion.

To a weeklong summer camp for teens in east Tennessee.

To Smith Lake, two hours south of us, several times over the summer.

To Point Mallard Water Park in Decatur, AL.

To Cathedral Caverns for the day.

To Nashville, TN, to see Shakespeare in the Park's rendition of *The Comedy of Errors*.

To attend a two-week family vacation to Crater Lake National Park; Bend, OR; Portland, OR; several stops down the Oregon Coast; and Redwoods National Park in northern California.

To Franklin, TN, for another soccer tournament.

To visit his aunt and uncle in Austin, TX, and go to Austin City Limits music festival.

To go camping at Buffalo Point Campground in the Buffalo National River Recreation Area.

To Chattanooga, TN, to a climbing gym for a birthday adventure.

To tour Vulcan Quarry for fossils in Falkville, AL.

To attend a four-day homeschool field trip to Dauphin Island Sea Lab.

To go hiking at High Point Falls south of us.

You can travel to do OIT, and you can travel while you do OIT!

If it was a longer trip, we had to plan a bit more. For both the week at camp and the family trip to the west coast, we had to make sure that we had an OIT updose appointment very close to the day we left so that as little time as possible went by before he could have another updosing appointment when he returned home. Sending Alex off to camp with his dosing required explaining the protocol to the camp director and camp nurses. They handled the dose each day like a medicine dose that he had to go to the nurse to get.

Alex had attended this camp for three years prior, and they were great with food allergies, keeping all meals served to campers nut free, doing vegetarian and vegan and celiac diets as well. They were amazing with accepting the reality of Alex's anaphylactic allergy AND accepting that now he was doing OIT to become desensitized, he had to eat x milligrams a day that looked like 1 peanut! The nurses gave him his dose in a private area after breakfast each day, and when there weren't physical activities planned for the mornings, he was monitored by them for the waiting period, and it worked without a hitch.

Anytime we had things coming up that would necessitate the dose being at a different time of day, we would slowly move the dose from afternoon to morning over the course of a few days, keeping it administered within the allergist's recommended window. For example, at camp, he needed to dose after breakfast so the week before camp, we slowly moved his dose to the morning one hour at a time earlier each day.

When the doses were solution, I took on the responsibility of helping to measure his dose and watch Alex administer every day. Since it was a liquid and new, it seemed a fragile science that I needed to oversee. When the doses got to actual peanut pieces, OIT picked up speed and integrated quickly into our day's routine.

If I wasn't present when he dosed, he would call or text me and say he was dosing. He measured out the doses for each week in a pill container. Initially, he used a stacked screw together one, and later a travel pill zipper case when the daily peanut count got higher than would fit in the other one. It was pre-measured weekly and separated out by each day. The allergist had given us a fine gram jewelry scale to measure peanuts for dosing. It lives in our kitchen on the coffee shelf. Just like the *EpiPen* and doses of antihistamine and antacid, the OIT dose pouch travelled with Alex everywhere so that he was ready to dose if his plans changed. He didn't keep his dose at home only.

Traveling TO OIT

I hate to drive. I will volunteer my car if someone else wants to drive it, or opt to be the passenger taking care of the kids rather than sit behind the wheel. It tires me visually and physically to drive. I have a benign tumor in my right knee that hasn't needed to be removed yet, but my leg seems to fatigue easier on long drives than it used to. I was not looking forward to the long drives there and back in a day for OIT, but in order to fit it into our family's full calendar, we often had to make the round trip in one day. It was the closest option. We wanted to do OIT, so we did it, but I had a lot of trepidation about the driving.

It turns out that driving to OIT every two weeks with Alex was the part of the OIT journey that I most treasure. I dreaded it for nothing. A couple of months into OIT, Alex got interested in driving. He had gotten his permit right before he turned sixteen the fall before, but had not been interested in driving. Once he got his permit, he took over some of the driving each time there and back and refined his driving skills along the way. He would have never had that much highway and interstate driving experience if it weren't for our trips to OIT sharing the wheel.

More than OIT being added driving time for a learning driver, it was hours of quality time that I would have never scheduled with my teen son. Having three other younger kids, something would have always interrupted us. Because of the time crunch of family life and the phase of life, how many teen boys spend hours in conversation and presence with their mom? We had some early morning drives that weren't fueled by much other than coffee and an interesting podcast to keep us awake. But we also had time to talk, time without eye contact.

I will treasure those drives with Alex for the rest of my life. Other than a handful of OIT office visits, I drove Alex to OIT instead of Kurt and arranged care for the other kids. We listened to the *Ready Player One* by Ernest Cline audiobook. He survived my obsession with the *Serial* and *Undisclosed* Podcasts. We listened to all the *Radiolabs* and many *This American Life* podcasts.

Over this time, Alex was also prepping to take the ACT. He had chunks of hours to use the ACT app while riding in the car on an iPad. While I wish and hope for others of you to have an OIT doctor as close to you as you can, in your town preferably, it was a bonus that we had to travel to do OIT. It gave me one-on-one time with my son. It gave me a down day in the busyness of life. We listened to things and learned and broadened our minds in those drives. This time together was the silver lining in having to travel to see a private practice OIT allergist.

Doing OIT with a kid while having three other kids is not for the faint. I put all my energy into making it work. I was drawing credit on all the future years I wouldn't have to put energy into avoiding peanuts like I always had. I did double duty to make the future easier. This meant prepping what my younger kids would eat ahead of time on the days I was gone and where they would be.

When we left for OIT, I called on family and friends for favors or paid baby sitters to watch my other kids. I treated this situation as if I worked one day a week. I essentially "worked" one day a week every other week as OIT transport service. The other three kids were either tagging along with Dad while he worked around town or from home, or they had all their needs met and a day planned for them in someone else's care.

Since we homeschool, the kids are always with one of us, usually me, so leaving them with someone else was a bit more of a feat. Since I was usually their parent, teacher, and driver to all classes and activities, we all had to make a big adjustment when I left for the day to an OIT appointment starting early in the morning. I could not have done this for Alex for eight months without the support and hands on help of my parents who were always there if we needed them; my sister who was available even with a baby under a year old to come be at my house in my place; and friends that took kids for the day either in my home, to their house, or even to Chattanooga one time; and my parents and aunt who did drove the kids around while I was gone. They all gave Alex the gift of OIT as much as anyone. It was an extended family and friend affair. I can't ever repay that kind of help, but I will pay it forward one day.

CHAPTER 15 - OIT WITH A TEEN

OIT with a teen is all I know. I didn't see many teens online in the groups doing OIT when I was researching. Nor did I hear of many teen patients doing OIT from the doctors we consulted. As there is more published online, I now know that it is more common than I thought. There is a whole section on the OIT101 website with teen and adult stories[8] of those who have undergone OIT. There is a kid to kid Facebook group[9] where kids who are doing or considering OIT can connect. Dr. Kari Nadeau says, "Everyone's immune system is capable of adapting, and surprisingly, it is as true of adults as children." (OIT101, 2016e)

Originally, I was perplexed why there were not more people Alex's age and more adults doing OIT. I feared it was more dangerous for older teens and adults, and that resulted in very few teens and adults doing OIT. Thus, I worried we were too late to help Alex through OIT. Those unfounded fears were all taken away at our consults. The allergist assured me it was not any different for Alex than for a younger child other than the difference in ability to communicate, be a part of the process, and understand OIT as an adult would.

The only theory that made sense was what one doctor offered. He thought that many older teens and adults have gotten used to avoidance; thus, it wasn't worth it to them to make the big time commitment from work or school to undergo OIT. He theorized that their motivations for a social and emotional cure were not as high as parents of younger kids who wanted the constraints of a food allergy solved for their kid's childhood. The theory was basically that these older allergic patients had perhaps gotten comfortable in their allergy avoidance life.

This was an interesting theory because this is exactly why I wanted Alex to do OIT: because he was leaving childhood and heading into adulthood where his food allergy life didn't seem comfortable or safe. To me as a parent of a teen with a food allergy, adulthood ahead seemed like a ballooning of risk factors that I was desperate to pop or contain as much as possible. OIT seemed perfectly suited to do this. A tool to get Alex through his young adult life safely.

I intuit that this dosing experience and this conquering experience with Alex's allergen is a different path than it would have been if he'd been a younger child. At the outset, he had to be all in. When I first wanted Alex to explore OIT and he was unwilling, it would have been counterproductive to force the issue. Since OIT doses needed to be calmly eaten daily, he had to be completely on board.

Manipulating or creatively getting him to take doses as a teen would have been a dynamic that wasn't possible due to his maturity and awareness nor would it have been peace giving to either of us. OIT wasn't required for him to survive like the *EpiPen* dose at a reaction. I desired OIT in our lives in order to make him safer all the time. Again, OIT felt proactive and not reactive, and it took some time to wrap Alex's head around that different approach to his allergy. With OIT, he could alter the effect of his food allergy on his life that he'd been told all along he had no control over.

We had those difficult conversations about the reality of his adult life ahead of him, avoiding food, and the life-threatening risks I feared for him. Those truthful, scary conversations were a part of the equation that ended in Alex agreeing to explore OIT. It was certainly not a decision that ever felt to him or to me like it was all roses. However, after he thought about it for a year, and he heard my true concern and rational plea to allow us to try and reverse the danger of peanuts by desensitizing his body, he got it and said yes. A younger Alex would have gone along with what mom suggested at the very beginning.

OIT with a teen is all I know, but I don't advocate waiting if you are considering Oral Immunotherapy unless your OIT allergist advises waiting for a reason. I wish Alex had been younger when I discovered OIT, and he agreed to do it. Mainly, so he could have been free from the fear and anxiety of an accidental ingestion and endured less social restriction when he was younger. And selfishly, just for me to have had more days and months and years of freedom from carrying the weight of fear and anxiety for my child.

If OIT had been on my radar ten years ago, and available, when Alex was seven, I would have been elated. I would have set that emotional burden of food allergy down at the first mention I'd heard that there was a possibility of doing so.

I imagine it would have been easier to do OIT if he were younger. I perceive that he would not have been as scared, as reluctant, as delayed in embracing it if I'd been able to simply explain it as a medicine to his younger self. At the same time, I think he has a grasp and a reverence for OIT and daily dosing because of his older age. I think he will always remember life and what it felt like before OIT gave him a measure of safety, control, and freedom with his peanut allergy.

Some allergists have been doing OIT for almost a decade in private practice, but not any of them are near us. I say that I would have been the first to do OIT if I knew about it ten years ago, but it would have been difficult. Traveling with a seven year old when I had two other children under the age of eight would have been more difficult. Even if I wanted it more than anything for Alex, it might have been near impossible to pull off. It was a collision of happenstance and courage that put it in his lap at age 16. We had an allergist not too far away. He was mature and able to understand the before and after and the process.

I don't doubt for a second that Alex will remember life before OIT and life after, and this will keep him diligent about dosing more than anything the allergist or science explain about the protocol. Being a young adult is a time in life that can be full of carelessness. I am glad he has this perspective on OIT to hold it in seriousness. In short, one benefit of him not getting to OIT until now is that he fully owns it. It's his decision, his hard work, his responsibility. But, I'd still do it earlier if I could!

Alex has been better about taking his daily OIT dose than I ever expected. He is not always particularly conscientious with regards to time or placement of things. In my experience with my four kids, some of us are born more organized and others of us must work hard at that part of fitting into the world. Alex has a lack of attention to detail at times, which can result in him leaving the house without his shoes on and not even notice until he is at his destination. This has even happened as a teen! He is a very spontaneous, creative, and carefree type of person. I often envy this in him. Alex is not a worrier at heart, which allows him to forget more things than a worrier like me does. Because my head is always plotting and planning and worrying ahead of time and it's exhausting, I see his lack of worry as a blessing.

However, this trait has also given him considerable frustration in his life. We try to help him not forget things by creating habits and processes to leave the house, but he still forgets sometimes. When he first started carrying his bag, *EpiPen*, water, and snacks when he left the house, it was a struggle to help him remember to have everything with him. Now as an older teen, after enough times of me driving him back home to get his *EpiPen* as a child, he finally remembers to bring everything. It is now ingrained. It finally stuck.

Knowing that, I wondered how we were going to get daily dosing to stick as well. I stressed over ways to get him in the mindset or tools he could have at his disposal to help him remember something so important. We have tried it all in attempting to make it a seamless part of life. Kurt, Alex, and I all put alarms on our phones. We put the OIT dosing stuff prominently on the kitchen island. When it was a struggle to remember, we experimented and brainstormed with Alex to determine what time of day worked best to tack on this OIT task, where it flowed and make sense, and when was it more likely for him to remember to dose.

This has been an important change in his life and the most important part of OIT to master. It has been as much of a milestone to celebrate, remembering to dose, as getting to his maintenance dose in December. In order to succeed and have Alex take full responsibility, taking his dose needed to become second nature. For a while, it felt like I had just replaced my fear and worry of Alex eating peanuts to worrying whether he remembered to dose. I didn't want to trade one lifetime worry for another, so handing this portion off to Alex was important to me for both of our sanities sake. This has been no easy feat for a teen that suffers from forgetfulness and has a fluctuating life schedule.

We tried the OIT dosing app someone created, and for a short while, that worked well in helping us keep track of things. But, what really worked was keeping it visual in the home and setting alarms. I am stunned to say that in Alex's whole eight months of daily dosing until he was on maintenance, he only forgot to take his dose one day. This missed dose was in the second half of his OIT journey when he was on higher gram doses of actual peanuts. We followed the allergist's order when it happened, and there were no reactions or ill side effects because of this mistake. And then once since graduation to maintenance, Alex missed a daily dose. Again, consultation with the allergist and following doctor's orders for the next dose worked. Mistakes will happen with daily dosing but so far they have been few and inconsequential.

I am concerned about him dosing every day for life. Right now, it is easy. Since he's here in my home, I can see if he took his dose or not by checking whether the pill container for that day is empty. He's seeing what dosing will be like for him as an adult. He prepares his own doses; he has a schedule now where he takes his dose with him if he leaves the house. It's been added to his *EpiPen* area of his bag, so a dose is always on hand no matter where he is when he doses.

However, for now, he has mom and dad reminding him. Most every day, I still check or ask him if he dosed that day. He has a younger sister that singsongs "OIT" with each syllable strung out for seconds as a silly reminder. She started months ago in the car overhearing a conversation we were having.

Like it is for anyone that takes medication, it's possible to make it second nature. I trust and know he will get there. It's a small price to pay, a daily ritual of eating peanuts, for a lifetime of freedom from the fear and anxiety. Initially, this fear that he wouldn't remember to dose assimilated into daily life for me, as tantamount to a panic about eating something with peanut at an event. But as time went on, it became a different, calmer level of concern.

I know now that a skipped dose can be handled with the allergist. I know now that many patients must skip doses during their protocol due to illness or other reasons, and then they pick it back up without affecting their progress or reactivity. It's ok for it to be a rare occurrence, and the panic at the rare occurrence of forgetting to dose is nothing compared to the panic at the rare occurrence of accidental ingestions in our pre-OIT lives.

When I'm not always there with Alex in the future, there will always be other friends and loved ones watching out for him. That's always been the case for every person in his life whom he is close to. He has had help regarding keeping him safe from peanuts. He will have support remembering to eat peanuts daily as he has support eradicating them daily in the past.

The research about continuing to need a daily dose with OIT is still ongoing. There is some hope that a daily dose may not be needed, and it can be scaled back to a weekly dose or less. "The patient completing the full OIT protocol does not have to add the food freely back into his/her diet, but the daily maintenance "dose" has to be ingested to maintain the desensitization. At this time, this is considered to be a lifetime protocol, much the same as taking a daily medication or even like daily hygiene routines such as brushing our teeth.

For some patients, in the future, they may not need to dose daily but a few times a week for a lifetime." According to Dr. Nadeau of Stanford[10]: "When the children's blood and skin-prick tests become negative to the allergens, which happens somewhere between six months and three years on the maintenance dose, Nadeau believes that a small amount of the allergens (for example, one peanut a day or the amount of egg and milk in one pancake) will be enough to prevent the allergy from returning" (OIT101, 2016f).

So, there is hope on the horizon for the daily dose to be scaled back in the future, but no certainty of this yet. Either way, to this mom and to my son, eating peanuts every day for life is far preferable to fearing peanuts every day for life.

CHAPTER 16 - GRADUATING TO MAINTENANCE

Gaining Confidence

While Alex's childhood was miraculously devoid of anxiety, it is clear to you by now that I did not dodge anxiety. I took anxiety and turned it into an illusion of control. There were so many things through the years that were what I call the "Neverland" of his childhood. Like the land in Peter Pan, this was a mythical place where children who were not food allergic experienced carefree things. Neverland was all the things that were never, ever going to be a part of our lives.

There were a mishmash of cultural things and food places he couldn't experience, moments that when taken individually don't matter, but when added up seem like Alex missed out on a normal childhood. But, did Alex miss them? No, I don't think that he did. Food allergy life itself can be made full. Alex had a temperament and circumstances that weathered it well. There are many grown adults with food allergies who feel they have full, thriving lives. It is

171

the emotional bits that I wish I could wave a wand over. The social awkwardness that exists.

While I cared about these things in Neverland that I put on a pedestal, Alex didn't care; he's told me as much, but I miss that he missed out on them. I would have liked to share the carefree with him back then when he was still little. Being on the other side of Oral Immunotherapy and being bite safe from peanuts now, there are things that jump out at me all the time and I realize, wow, we never did that ever! These are the things that I protected that I realize now he could have had in his childhood if he'd either not been allergic to peanuts or if we'd known about and could do Oral Immunotherapy earlier in his life.

I didn't realize how boxed in we were until we stepped outside that reality and the walls I'd created for 16 years. Alex didn't do so many minor, irrelevant things. Again, they truly appear to not matter to him, and they matter little compared to so many other difficulties in the world at large. I wonder though, don't they matter when piled up cumulatively? Yes, in my opinion, they do.

The combined effect of tiptoeing around different food situations, living in hesitation, and always waiting for the next shoe of contamination to drop, that matters. Living in the position of half-heartedly having to trust the world at large regarding food safety, all while knowing logically and rationally that you couldn't trust the world at large when it came to your food allergy ever, that matters.

Living knowing one day a reaction will happen, either by your fault or someone else's, this matters. Most likely an innocuous reason, contamination, or bad labeling would cause the reaction, but it would require an *EpiPen*. Hopefully, the *EpiPen* would be on hand as planned and everything would be ok like the other five times. But it's the reality that, once again, my child stood unwillingly on that cliff teetering on the edge of his life, out of control, at the mercy of the cocktail made between his accidental ingestion, his body's systems and epinephrine. Epinephrine is a wonder drug, but it must be given in time to work, so a reaction must be noticed and given serious attention within an unknown window of time. So many gears must fall into place to turn the wheel in your favor.

Living in that box, Alex and I were used to lowering our excitement and confidence. Life outside our home or around others, especially when food or snacks came up, was only experienced in a wary state. Food avoidance kept everything in life a little clouded. It was glorious over those eight months in OIT to take steps out of that fog.

One day during OIT, our foggy state must have been very apparent. We hadn't been in a Chick-Fil-A since the early 2000s. And when we visited again, their menu had changed. Five of us stood there at the counter and tried to decipher the menu. I could tell this Chick-Fil-A didn't get a lot of first time visitors. Their normal customers have slowly adapted to their menu changes over the past 15 years and don't stand at the counter like they are reading a foreign film's subtitles.

After we studied the menu and each decided on our order, we stepped up to the counter. As the cashier was getting us our beverages, I sensed she was focusing on me a bit more than normal. Finally, unable to contain her curiosity, she said as she handed me our last drink, "Y'all aren't from around here are you?"

Surprised, and not sure where she was going with this and feeling a little creeped out that she knew we were traveling, I thought a second and said, "No, we are not."

She then asked, "Where are you from?"

I think she was sorely disappointed in my answer when I said "We are from a few hours north" because she slightly furrowed her eyebrows and said, "Oh."

I wish I'd thought to ask why she asked me, but I think I know. Only a family from another country or another part of the country or world could be such novices ordering at a Chick-Fil-A counter. We were newly moved in from the planet of peanut allergy avoidance. Yes, we appear odd because we are aliens here on this new surface where peanuts are no longer a danger. That's how alien we looked, pegged as international travelers in our state capital. This experience pretty much sums up what it's like to walk outside of the restrictions you had before OIT. Life without fear of peanut avoidance and cross contamination is a whole new planet. It's so clear when you are out of the fog how hard it was to see.

Freedom from the stress of food allergy avoidance happened in little moments. In time, confidence replaced the stress, worry, and anxiety. When you are not burdened with worry and anxiety, self-confidence can blossom. Minor events felt like fireworks, celebratory little mini parties of freedom. Sometimes, it was apparent as I would cry in an instant, great big, silent dripping tears of relief. Other times it was hidden from view in order to not embarrass my son, who doesn't outwardly share the same level of relief I do at the freedom of OIT.

Over these eight months and after OIT graduation to maintenance, I attribute this new OIT confidence in giving Alex the ability to step out and do things that until this point, he'd kept on the back burner. For example, he decided he wanted to drive after two years of no interest in the task whatsoever. I know other teens these days who are not as eager to drive. I think this is because there are many ways for teens to connect virtually with friends and groups and events, but Alex's reluctance didn't ever fully make sense to me. He is one of my extroverted kids. I thought he would want to get behind a wheel as soon as he could and drive himself to places he wanted to be without counting on me. But he had not wanted to.

Likely, feeling like he couldn't trust the world to keep him safe, and being in it completely alone in a car was too much to hurdle if he didn't have to. Five months into OIT, after many miles of driving during our trips to updose appointments, he out of the blue said he wanted to go test for his license. When I asked him what caused him to change his mind, my caring child said, "I think it would be nice for you to not have to take me where I want to go anymore." His change of heart was about having confidence to take the responsibility of his transport and safety off me and onto himself. I think his change of heart was made possible as his load of fear and worry about being safe lightened and confidence stepped in.

As my fear of peanuts was whittled down over the OIT process, I then began to worry about having a driving teenager. In those early months of him driving, I worried like the peanut worry, life and death. He was at the mercy of his abilities, other strangers' abilities, weather patterns, and flukes like animals darting into the road.

After feeling a life and death worry for 16 years, it was grand to only feel it in small bursts while he was a new driver. And my worry over him driving diminished each time he drove. I didn't realize the feeling of the latent fear, until it had been fading, and then I suddenly felt it course through my body again as he drove off for the first time. It was nice to know my worry of him driving would have a more finite end and my body would assimilate back to a stress-free state.

Shedding Stress

At every updose visit, I gained more confidence in OIT, recognizing its life-saving impact, both soul and emotion. The relief was so profound at the fear I didn't have to carry anymore: he was eating peanuts. I could now set down my fear that Alex might have a fatal accidental ingestion that wouldn't be noticed by him or others in time. Through tears, I released the stress I had been holding.

I also cried for those who still carry a life-threatening food allergy burden; for those who don't get to feel this free because they don't know of OIT yet, or don't trust it will work for them, or have an inability to get to the end. I cried for those who have already lost their loved ones, those who OIT might have been able to protect. I cried for the ten percent for whom OIT won't succeed because of the particulars of their allergies and conditions and ability to comply.

I cried at the idea of this humble doctor who has no family with life-threatening food allergies of his own, nor any food allergies himself, stepping out on a limb by offering Oral Immunotherapy and changing kids' lives. I held back at each updose, but I felt each time like tackling him with a hug, squeezing him tight, and thanking him profusely. I did thank him sincerely each time, but in a more professional manner. I got teary in front of our allergist at Alex's second to last visit. I just couldn't believe Alex only had one more visit and only saying thank you felt so paltry and insignificant.

I joked that I wanted to buy him a car or a house or a life changing vacation around the world, but that honestly nothing I could say or do could ever thank him enough. He heard me, but I don't think he will ever understand the hero he and his nurse are to me. I can't see the screen as I type this because every time that I think of it consciously, the tears stream down my face. Sitting here in a coffee shop, listening to headphones while typing out different combinations of the 26 letters of the alphabet in a feeble attempt to describe this relief from OIT, I am aware that everyone around me likely thinks I am reading news of a loved one's death rather than recording my son's new life free from peanut doom. I've got sixteen years of tears to cry out. It's going to be a while before I stop; I've got more cries left inside of me before I let that old peanut crazed mother in me go.

I remember my first big meltdown. It was the week before Halloween this past year. I used to hold my breath from October through March when it finally warmed up, and we were out of the high red alert stage 10 danger zone of the food infested holidays. Alex also has pollen allergies that are worse in the fall, so it always seemed like his system was a bit overloaded in these months. Incidentally all his anaphylactic reactions, except the first, happened between October and March when it got warm again.

My first meltdown happened when Alex attended our city's teen costume ball, which he has for several years. It was held at the large main public library, from 8pm to midnight, with no adults allowed. A DJ music pumped dance party, with cosplay and creativity fueled by teens. He loved it. But it was exactly the type of event that put me in knots: he was alone, revelry as a focus instead of diligence, loud music, a room of snacks and candy, dancing, potential sharing of drinks, etc. The list of worries was usually long.

There were a multitude of scary scenarios that played out in my subconscious at an event like this. Dancing at that level could exacerbate an allergic symptom or mask an allergic symptom. I took him and dropped him off each year. I embraced it, but honestly every fiber in my body was tense the entire time. No one was watching out for him except himself. I wondered how watchful he would be in this party state that was not a nut free environment.

After reminding Alex to be peanut aware at the ball and dropping him off, I packed up and internalized my fear. I simply gave him an upbeat verbal warning and kept him moving on happily forward, as I always did.

I had chosen not to keep him in a bubble, with the exception of deciding to homeschool him to keep him safe. Even after he reacted to curry that one time, I still allowed him to try to make a food situation safe if he wanted, instead of keeping some foods homemade only.

But, just because I let him go doesn't mean I could easily let the fear go. Every bubble wrap free moment was filled with guilt and fear. Sending him off to week long camp felt like this. Sending him off for two weeks with his grandparents felt like this. The costume ball felt like this.

He had been gone from the house for about three hours, and I hadn't thought once about him being away at the ball other than watching the clock for pickup time. He was going with a large group of teens to Waffle House for after midnight breakfast, and I was one of the drivers.

My phone chimed on the kitchen counter with an alert that I had a message. It was my daughter sending me a picture from the ball, telling me they had met up with the new friend that was coming to meet the group. After texting her back, thanking her for looking out for the new friend, I walked into my room and it hit me like a thunderstorm: until I got that text, I hadn't thought about Alex's safety at the ball.

It was the first time he had been away, and I had not thought frequently of his safety. He had been at an event filled with plenty of risk for several hours, and I didn't worry or let anxiety consume me. I fell into a sobbing mess on my bed. I called Kurt, who was at work, and sobbed tears of joy and relief on the phone.

Alex was away, and he was safer than he'd ever been. He was free from cross contamination and contact danger at the amount he was eating now, and likely somewhat bite safe. I fully realized in that moment what OIT was going to give him and us. That night, fear free allergy life was birthed as I sobbed on the phone with Kurt.

These were not tame tears running down my cheeks these were full body sobs, trembling with joy, relief, gratitude and hope that I never thought could be ours. Freedom from the fear of this peanut allergy was going to be amazing. I locked myself in the bathroom as I didn't want my two younger kids to see me. They wouldn't understand mom in this sobbing state. I had always held this peanut mess so neatly for everyone, so emotionally healthy on the outside. My insides were showing. This weeping human in front of them would be too much.

Be prepared that if you undergo OIT for yourself or your child, and you've held onto worry and anxiety for any years, you might cry buckets of tears. You might do this multiple times especially if you have a child that lived a lot of their life with a food allergy. Be prepared to bawl; they need to add that to the OIT preparation materials. As of this writing, I've had two more big crying sessions since that ball. Each time sheds a little more of those sixteen years of stress. I suspect I've got a good cry in me for each year of Alex's life before OIT, so only thirteen more cries to go!

CHAPTER 17 - LIFE AFTER OIT

Alex had his last updose appointment on December 28, 2016. He is in "maintenance mode" for a year or less. After that point, with labs and a food challenge, he could graduate to being able to freely eat and add peanuts in his diet. If Alex passes this larger food challenge, it will mean that he can freely eat peanuts if he wants. He will still take his daily dose to stay desensitized until the research advises otherwise, but he will also be able to eat a Reese's peanut butter cup if he wants, or a Girl Scout tag-a-long cookie. His current maintenance level makes him bite safe and cross contamination safe, releasing the fear of an anaphylactic reaction. The next level of graduation could give him complete freedom to eat his allergen at will, above and beyond the tolerance or maintenance dose of eight peanuts.

Each day that we walk further from his last appointment seems like weeks away from the fear filled life I lived before the freedom of OIT. I wonder, even though Alex lived allergic without the social and emotional cure of OIT for sixteen years, how much he will remember the full impact of his allergy. I think his memory of the anaphylactic reactions will keep him dosing, but I am not certain he is holding onto any of the other mental impacts. OIT is painting thick strokes of positivity over all the negative, heavy emotions of living with the allergy.

Oral Immunotherapy has left him in such a thriving state, so I'm not certain he will remember much about being deeply fearful of peanuts. Starting at age 17, this past fall, he was eating a handful of peanuts every day. I no longer fear the pile of peanuts in his cup. Will his body, head, and heart remember what it felt like before to see peanuts? Or will his brain rewrite that past emotional history and help him see peanuts like a medicine that he takes to stay out of danger, like an aspirin a day for heart health in an at-risk patient?

I think I'll remember fear a lot longer and feel its impact longer than Alex will. Alex has always taken his food allergy as a matter of fact, carried it in stride. I always took it as a huge crater in our life and in my heart, even though I hid that crater. In this regard, OIT has been catastrophe reversing for me.

Two months out, I am still in excitement mode; in contrast, my teen son is very chill with his new normal. When I question his lack of excitement, he says, "It's normal, Mom; this is what OIT said it would provide; this is what I expected so it's not surprising. There isn't a reason to freak out or make a big deal." He hasn't shed a tear yet in joy or in relief to my knowledge. Maybe he still will one day. Maybe he just never viewed life as lacking as I thought he did, maybe he wasn't holding the stress of avoidance as close to his heart. If so, that means I did well: he felt a childhood of abundance, and not fear, despite his allergy.

For Alex, his maintenance dose is seven grams. In Whole Foods brand unsalted roasted peanuts, which run on the smaller side, this varies anywhere from seven to nine peanuts. The peanut maintenance dose might be different for each patient, again OIT is individualized. It also looks and progresses and ends drastically different depending on the allergen that is being desensitized. I'm sharing Alex's peanut daily dose amount here, while I have otherwise intentionally left out the updose and amount specifics of his OIT experience, so you can visualize what Alex eats everyday now. This is not to be taken as a "how to" reference or for anyone else to compare their OIT journey with peanuts to Alex's journey. Low dosage and slower time in OIT is a valid and celebrated outcome as well. If you embark on peanut OIT or OIT for any other allergen and your journey looks different than this, you have still succeeded in conquering an allergen!

I've shared my story to spread the news, to give perspective on a life before and after a food allergy using Oral Immunotherapy. Nothing in this story is meant to be used as a substitute for consultation about a food allergy or any other medical condition with your doctor, a board-certified allergist you trust or a board certified OIT allergist. This is a heart share, not a medical share.

Alex is 6-12 months out from his final "challenge" later in 2017 to see if he can tolerate free eating peanuts. He will stay on his daily maintenance dose even if he passes that challenge unless his allergist advises an altered dosing schedule. I am beyond thrilled to know that research shows it is possible Alex will not pass food allergy genes on to his children. It has been the part of his peanut allergy that I wish I could take back, any effect that my genes and Kurt's genes had on Alex developing his allergy. To know he likely won't pass a genetic predisposition to peanut allergy on to his children is the next best thing. (OIT101, 2016g)

Finally feeling the warmth of the sun after Alex's last appointment, the light at the end of the tunnel, had me exuberant on our drive home. It was hard to sit still but we had to get back home. I asked Alex if I could roll down the windows and sunroof as it was a mild December day. He obliged. I then glanced over at him driving and asked if I could scream without scaring him while he was driving.

"No, Mom, someone will hear you and worry about us!"

"No, they won't," I countered, "it'll be a scream of joy."

"I don't get why, Mom, that's really weird."

"It's just so exciting for me, Alex, to be done with updosing and realize that it means that you and I can live not afraid anymore. I have lived afraid for so long."

Alex did not relent, so instead, I did a muffled scream seventeen times. It sounded like the amplified squeak of a mouse. An anticlimactic "eeeep" noise that stood in for the feeling I had. I felt we were being released from sixteen years of peanut prison, wrongfully convicted and with our sentences fully served. One squeak of joy escaped me for each year. Alex rolled his eyes and gave me a big smile as he drove us home.

That's our story of crushing the peanut. After trying futilely for sixteen years to subdue and suppress food allergy's hold on Alex's life and my heart and head, we conquered. This nut, shell and all, is destroyed, an enemy no more. Slowly at first with peanuts pulverized into flour and swallowed in liquid like medicine and then later bravely with peanuts ground into crumbs by his own teeth, Alex literally crushed the allergic effect of peanuts on his body and life. My son will now live what I like to call "happily ever allergic." Food allergy diagnosis in our family is forever stripped of its fear and impact thanks to the desensitization of Oral Immunotherapy.

If you found _Crushing the Peanut_ inspiring or informative, please consider sharing the news of OIT with someone you know that has a life-threatening food allergy. Share my story and let them know about the website www.oit101.org.

If you can take a moment to leave me a REVIEW on Amazon.com, I greatly appreciate it. Thank you for helping spread the word about Oral Immunotherapy.

ACKNOWLEDGMENTS

To Alex, thank you for giving me permission to share your food allergy story out loud. I'm grateful to experience peanut allergy with you: a beautiful mess with an ending I couldn't imagine, and a ride I wouldn't have missed. I hope you can understand and forgive all my crazy parts. Your bravery to try OIT was a gift to you, and all of us who love and have protected you. I know it will be a gift to some reader affected by food allergy whom you don't even know. Thanks for this hope. I love you, and I love that you are safe.

To Kurt, Emma, Owen and Inde, love and thanks to you for the hours you put into this story, both through the years in our family as Alex's dad, sisters and brother, always being an advocate for Alex to live a full life; in this past year with your time and sacrifice to get him OIT treatment; and in the past few months when I put other parts of our lives on the back burner to get this story out of my head and into this narrative.

To my parents, Bill and Pam; sisters, Libby and Maggie; Aunt Patti; brother-in-laws, Michael and Jace; and extended family and friends. You all are a big part of the reason Alex got safely to 16 and got to crush this peanut allergy with Oral Immunotherapy! Without your support and care over his lifetime, he would not have been as safe, felt as included and accommodated, or been as full of confidence to undertake this. Thank you for honoring and respecting and treating his allergy as if it was one of your own. You made living with food allergies in community as painless as it could be. Not everyone has such a large group helping them keep their food allergic child safe. I did have a large group of helpers that went above and beyond. An army. Everyone one of you that made your homes and your gatherings peanut safe and life inclusive for Alex for the past sixteen years are a hidden hero in this story. I understand what you gave and did and I am forever thankful.

To Dr. A and Danielle, there aren't adequate words. Thank you for giving food allergy patients hope and lives without fear and stress instead of just counseling them on food avoidance. "Dr. A," Dr. Ruchir Agrawal, Alex's allergist, is a board-certified allergy and immunology physician at Freedom Allergy, located in Peachtree City and Marietta, Georgia. He provides personalized care to patients with severe asthma, food allergies, environmental allergies, allergic rhinitis, and any related allergic disorders. He also specializes in food allergies and offers oral immunotherapy (OIT) for patients with peanut, tree nut, milk, and egg allergies. Freedom Allergy aims to equip all patients with the necessary information and treatments to enjoy a life free of asthma and allergy symptoms. That bio is just a long way of saying visit Freedom Allergy, OIT is their game, Superheroes are their name!

To Liseetsa Mann, Gail Reynolds Frank, Donna Lin Chen and the hundreds of other food allergy parents who made the OIT communities come alive online for me and who came to my rescue with just the right word or the right resource when I was searching and scared. Thank you for making those safe places to walk through OIT as informed and supported as I could be. You are changing the face of food allergy.

And to my handful of helpers and inspirers on this project, my first book. A thank you goes to Ramy Vance for coaching and deadlines and to Lisa Weber for pointing out last summer the fun game that writing could be. I am grateful for being gifted the Self-Publishing School Course that gave me a blueprint for writing this book. I am indebted to my volunteer OIT ambassador team that helped me spread this story. Thank you all for contributing to my first book experience. Now that I have this real-life journey recorded, my fingers and brain are free and ready for fiction!

REFERENCES

Crawford, E. (2005). Roamschool. Retrieved January, 2017, from www.roamschool.com

Food Allergy Research & Education. (n.d.). Retrieved January, 2017, from https://www.foodallergy.org/

Fraser, H. A. (2011). *The Peanut Allergy Epidemic: What's Causing it and How to Stop it.* New York, NY: Skyhorse Pub.

Mayer, C. (2012). OIT Center. Retrieved January, 2017, from http://www.oitcenter.com/

National Institute of Allergy and Infectious Disease. (2017, January). Addendum Guidelines for the Prevention of Peanut Allergy in the United States: Summary for Parents and Caregivers. Retrieved January, 2017, from

https://www.niaid.nih.gov/sites/default/files/peanut-allergy-prevention-guidelines-parent-summary.pdf

OIT101. (2016a). TREATING FOOD ALLERGIES WITH ORAL IMMUNOTHERAPY. Retrieved January, 2017, from

http://www.oit101.org/

OIT101. (2016b). New York Times Magazine: Article on Dr. Nadeau and OIT. Retrieved January, 2017, from

http://www.oit101.org/research/new-york-times-magazine-article-on-dr-nadeau-and-oit/

OIT101. (2016c). Top 10 OIT Myths. Retrieved February 03, 2017, from http://www.oit101.org/top-10-oit-myths/

OIT101. (2016d). Starting doses and "threshold of tolerance". Retrieved January, 2017, from

http://www.oit101.org/research/starting-doses-and-threshold-of-tolerance/

OIT101. (2016e). Adult/Teen OIT Success Stories. Retrieved January, 2017, from http://www.oit101.org/adult-oit-success-stories/

OIT101. (2016f). FAQs / Q&A. Retrieved January, 2017, from http://www.oit101.org/faqs/#

OIT101. (2016g). New York Times Magazine: Article on Dr. Nadeau and OIT. Retrieved January, 2017, from

http://www.oit101.org/research/new-york-times-magazine-article-on-dr-nadeau-and-oit/

Peanut Component Panel. (2000). Retrieved January, 2017, from http://www.questdiagnostics.com/testcenter/TestDetail.action?ntc=9 1681

ENDNOTES

1 http://www.oit101.org/

2 https://www.facebook.com/groups/OIT101/

3 https://www.facebook.com/groups/PrivatePracticeOIT/

4 https://www.facebook.com/groups/OITCanada/

5 https://www.facebook.com/groups/OITUK/

6 https://www.facebook.com/groups/OITAustralia/

7 http://www.oitcenter.com/

8 http://www.oit101.org/adult-oit-success-stories/

9 https://www.facebook.com/groups/513896828749573/

10 http://www.oit101.org/research/new-york-times-magazine-article-on-dr-nadeau-and-oit/

42576794R00118

Made in the USA
Middletown, DE
15 April 2019